VITAMINS

What They Are and How They Can Benefit You

VITAMINS

What They Are and
How They Can Benefit You

BY HENRY BORSOOK, Ph.D., M.D.

Professor of Biochemistry, California Institute of Technology

New York

THE VIKING PRESS

1941

Second Printing December 1940
Third Printing January 1941

Foreword

DURING the past few years the public has become decidedly "vitamin-conscious." But, as so often happens, a new word has come into the common vocabulary without bringing with it any very clear understanding of what it means or of the importance of the developments which it represents.

The fact is that the discovery of the vitamins and of the role they play in human health is the most important medical advance so far made in this century. It has taught us what the essentials are in food. It has given us new insights into the chemistry of the body. But most important, it has given us the means of greatly raising the standard of health and well-being for all of us.

So far, we have barely begun to use this new knowledge. Measures have been taken to cure the diseases that result from diets gravely deficient in one or another of the vitamins. But, except for pellagra in the South, the severe vitamin-deficiency diseases are not a serious problem in the United States.

The really serious problem is that the general level of health is lower than it needs to be. Defective vision in dim light, most constipation and dyspepsia, the miscellaneous minor aches and pains of middle age, poor teeth, thinning of the bones, general fatigue and tonelessness—these are all very often caused by inadequate amounts of vitamins in our ordinary diets over a period of many years. In fact, what most of us consider normally good health is actually only mediocre health.

For the great majority of us, "buoyant" health—the sense of physical fitness, of being equal to the demands of daily life and work—can be attained by applying the present available knowledge of vitamins to ordinary diet. (Of course, in some cases, additional measures may be called for.) What is necessary is to get this knowledge of vitamins, with its technical jargon, assimilated into our everyday knowledge.

During the past half-dozen years I have been lecturing on vitamins to a wide variety of audiences—the general public, physicians, health officers, nurses, teachers, and dietitians. Invariably at the close of each lecture the audience wanted to know whether they could find anywhere a book containing all this information—as one of them put it, "in edible form."

The following pages are an attempt to supply such a book. For the men and women who want to know the facts for themselves and apply them to their own needs, its general information can be absorbed at a reading and it can be kept on hand for convenient reference. For the housewife (as well as the practicing physician, the nurse, and the dietitian) it should serve as a handbook of vitamin information which can be used as a cookery book is used, to plan the family meals.

Chapters I to XII are a kind of Cook's tour of the vitamins, explaining what they are, what they do, and where they are to be found. The tables which follow condense the essential information for practical day-to-day use. In applying this information to the planning of meals a little arithmetic is necessary—not more than ten or fifteen minutes on two or three occasions. This task is made simpler, I hope, by the examples of a day's food for children and adults (pages 167 to 176). But the task of a little arithmetic is a small price to pay for improving your general health and assuring your children a better physical start in life.

Since this discussion of vitamins is planned primarily for the general reader, I have omitted the technical details and minutiae of proof which would be required if it had been written for professional students and workers in the field of nutrition.

I wish to thank Mr. Upton Sinclair for his interest in this little book and for his help, and Mr. J. B. Hatcher, Research Assistant in Biochemistry at the California Institute of Technology, for bringing up to date the tables on pages 179 to 193.

I wish to thank especially my colleague, Professor William Huse, for his invaluable assistance in revising the manuscript and preparing it for publication.

H. Borsook

Pasadena, California
September 22, 1940

Contents

VITAMINS

What They Are and How They Can Benefit You

CHAPTER I

Introducing Vitamins

UNTIL a generation ago diet was a hit-and-miss affair. The author recalls when he was a medical student the warning of the professor of pediatrics that the immutable laws of infant feeding went through a complete cycle about every ten years. Theories about the diet of adults were almost as variable.

Under those circumstances the physician was the slave of his own temperament. He was either enthusiastic about the latest fads, some of which he invented himself; or he believed that the food that gave indigestion to our sturdy pioneering ancestors was good enough for us.

His attitude and practice gravitated toward either of two extremes. The first extreme is caricatured in Molière's *The Physician in Spite of Himself (Le Médecin malgré lui)*. The leading character of the play is Sganarelle, an ignorant but shrewd and impudent fagot-binder. Having to choose between taking a beating and representing himself as a very skillful physician, which he is not at all, he prefers to go through with the imposture. He throws himself into the role enthusiastically.

The scene is in the home of a girl who is feigning dumbness. Sganarelle is explaining to the father the nature of his daughter's malady.

SGANARELLE: *Thus these vapors which I speak of, passing from the left side, where the liver is, to the right side, where we find the heart, it so happens that the lungs having communication with the brain, meet in their course the said vapors . . . and because the said vapors . . . are endowed with a certain malignity . . . caused by the sharpness of these humors engendered by the concavity of the diaphragm . . . that is the precise reason that your daughter is dumb.*

THE FATHER: *It is undoubtedly impossible to argue better. There is but one thing that I cannot exactly make out: that is the whereabouts of the liver and the heart. It appears to me that you place them differently from what they are; the heart is surely on the left side and the liver on the right.*

SGANARELLE: *Yes; this was so formerly; but we have changed all that, and we nowadays practice the art on an entirely new system.*

In contrast with the faddist or charlatan is the other extreme type of physician. He refuses to have anything to do with newfangled notions. What he learned in medical school is the bedrock of truth. He is never worried; he is always sure of himself. He is represented in this very old medical story:

The patient says: "Doctor, are you sure of the diagnosis? A friend of mine was diagnosed as having pneumonia and she died of typhoid fever."

The doctor replies: "Madam, you may rest assured. When I treat a patient for pneumonia he dies of pneumonia."

Much of the eagerness of the faddist, as well as the reluctance of the conservative, to try new dietary theories can be attributed to the fact that until recently the scientific information available was inadequate. A few years ago in constructing a diet on scientific principles the physician took into account only three items: calories, protein, and some fresh fruit and vegetables to prevent scurvy. Today, a scientific analysis (for practical purposes) breaks diet down into at least eleven components: calories, protein, calcium, phosphorus, iron, and six (of the ten known) vitamins. Of these the vitamins are, from the practical point of view and from the point of view of understanding the chemical basis of vital processes, the most important.

Our knowledge of vitamins is comparatively recent. It goes back hardly more than a generation, and the most significant discoveries about their essential role in human well-being have been made in the last decade. This new knowledge enables us, in the words of Sganarelle, to "practice the art [of nutrition] on an entirely new system." The progress in the science of nutrition is not the substitution of new dogma and fad for old. The old facts are still facts. But the development of our knowledge of vitamins especially has so shifted the emphasis regarding what is most important that this change is tantamount to a revolution. To this extent, then, "we nowadays practice the art [of nutrition] on an entirely new system."

The history of our increase in knowledge of vitamins is too complicated to set down in detail here. It has grown out of the investigations of a very large number of research workers all over the civilized world; and progress has been due not so much to a few outstanding discoveries as to a great number of advances small in themselves but impressive in their total results.

There has long been evidence available of the connection between various diseases and deficiencies in diet. Scurvy, for instance, was for centuries the curse of long sea voyages, where the mariners' food was the traditional salt meat and hardtack. In the eighteenth century, as the records of the British Navy show, this limited diet was found to be the cause of the disease, and a cure was discovered in the addition of citrus fruit and vegetables. Such clues as this, however, which we see today as pointing directly to the existence of vitamins, were not then followed up in any profitable direction, probably because general ideas of nutrition were themselves not sufficiently advanced.

It was not, in fact, until 1881 that the first clear experimental evidence was produced for the existence of such dietary factors as we now call vitamins. In that year an investigator fed mice on an artificial mixture of all the then known constituents of milk—proteins, fats, carbohydrates, and salts. When the mice failed to survive on this mixture, he concluded that "a natural food such as milk must therefore contain besides these known principal ingredients small quantities of unknown substances essential to life."

For various reasons his work remained virtually unnoticed. Nevertheless, his phrase, "small quantities of unknown substances essential to life," states the fundamental concept. It was only after other workers arrived at the same concept—which they did from 1906 to 1910—that real progress in knowledge of vitamins began.

The name *vitamins* is a slight modification of a term invented in 1913. Up to that time the phrase "accessory food substances" had been commonly used to designate the "small quantities of unknown substances essential to life." In 1913 an investigator who believed that he had isolated one of these gave it the name *vitamine*. The prefix *vita* (the Latin word for *life*) was chosen to suggest the importance of these substances to life itself. The last part of the word, *amine*, is the name of a group of chemical compounds to which he thought all such substances belonged. This supposition later proved to be wrong, but by that time the word was already in wide use, since it provided a much-needed general designation. Rather than sacrifice such a convenient term the final *e* was dropped to prevent the mistaken chemical identification, and the word *vitamin* is now established in scientific literature and general use.

Vitamins can still be accurately described by the 1881 phrase, if one word of it is omitted. They are "small quantities of . . . substances essential to life." They are no longer unknown; they are no longer mysterious substances endowed with magical properties. The exact chemical nature of most of them has been established: they are for the most part simple chemicals. Seven of them are now manufactured commercially and sold in pure concentrated form over the counter. The part they play in the economy of the body—their function in preventing and curing disease and in maintaining a high level of health—has been demonstrated beyond question. As time goes on, further research will undoubtedly add to the number of vitamins and give us a fuller insight into the role they play in the chemistry of the body. But the information available about them today is ample to show that knowledge of the vitamins must occupy the same central position in nutrition that bacteriology does in sanitation and hygiene.

But this may not seem to answer the question: How is a vitamin to be defined?

Vitamins are chemical substances. One precise definition uses the language of chemistry, listing the elements of which the substance is composed, the proportions in which those elements occur, and their groupings. Thus vitamin C is $C_6H_8O_6$. The grouping of these elements is indicated by the name 2,3-dienol-*l*-gulonic acid lactone. But such a definition does not tell anyone except an organic chemist what the stuff is really like. The clue to the difficulty lies in the word "like." When we form a conception of something new to us, we tend to do so largely in terms of its similarity and dissimilarity to something with which we are already familiar. Vitamin C happens to be somewhat "like" sugar. Like sugar, the pure vitamin is white and of crystalline form. Like sugar, it has a definite taste, though it happens to be slightly bitter instead of sweet. Like sugar, it is a relatively simple chemical substance.

But nobody except chemists ever bothers about an accurate —that is, a chemical—definition of sugar. (And even such a definition tells us nothing about its physiological and psychological effects.) We all know what sugar is. We get it from sugar cane or sugar beets. It has various properties that differentiate it from other things in similar form, like salt and borax. And we use it in comparatively large amounts to sweeten things. It is so familiar a part of everyday life that for practical purposes we are content to think of it in terms that describe it without understanding what it essentially is or essentially does.

Similarly, for practical purposes we can best understand vitamins by such descriptive details as where they occur, their comparison with other substances which, like them, are necessary for life, and the purposes they serve in the body.

Vitamins have two characteristics which set them apart from the other substances the body uses. The first is the very small amount of them which is necessary to preserve health. When bacteria were first discovered, people were amazed at the smallness of the organisms which could do so much harm. Today we are similarly amazed at the smallness of the amount of vitamins which can do so much good. If one could isolate the daily intake of vitamins in a good diet, altogether they would appear only as a few grains of sugar and sand. Yet these few specks are essential to health, even to life. This is clearly shown in the following examples. One of the first diseases to be identified as a vitamin-deficiency disease was beri-beri or polyneuritis. In this disease there is crippling neuritis, the heart is affected, and there may be paralysis. Beri-beri is prevalent in the Far East and wherever polished rice is the principal item in the diet. Yet beri-beri can be prevented by consumption of 1/30,000 of an ounce of vitamin B_1 daily. One ounce of vitamin B_1 will supply eighty people for one year.

Another example is rickets. This disease results from a deficiency of vitamin D. Bowlegs, knock-knees, and much of the bad posture of adults are the sequels of rickets in childhood. One ounce of vitamin D will prevent the disease in eight hundred children for a year.

The second characteristic of vitamins as a group is the inability of the human body to make them. A few animals have the fortunate faculty of making one vitamin, but human beings must depend for their vitamin supply on sources outside themselves. For the most part, vitamins are formed by green plants on land and by algae and other smaller organisms in the sea. Until fairly recently, then, human beings had to secure their necessary vitamins directly from plants or indirectly from supplies stored in the flesh of various animals.

In the past few years, however, the synthesis of vitamins—that is, their artificial manufacture—has been progressing rapidly; and it is certain that others will soon be added to the seven that are now being produced commercially. It is worth while to stress the significance of the word "manufacture" as applied to vitamins. Vitamins are naturally occurring substances; ordinarily they are obtained from the food we eat. When they are manufactured, they are "made" in the same sense that dyes, rayon, and plastics are made. In the manufacture of vitamins, the factory may eventually supplant agriculture as the principal source of essential dietary factors, just as the chemical factories today are supplanting natural silk and cotton by the synthetics rayon and nylon.

Even now it is cheaper to manufacture a number of vitamins than to grow plants for the same purpose. While naturally occurring foods will continue for a long time to be the main source of vitamins for us human animals, the synthesized vitamins are invaluable in treating vitamin-deficiency diseases and in supplementing diets that furnish an inadequate supply of one or more of the necessary vitamins. Incidentally, vitamin synthesis has already developed important new branches of industry as a result of research which began purely as physiological and medical investigations; and these developments are only the beginning of a great biotechnology of the future.

Besides knowledge of the nature of the vitamins themselves, research in the last decade has given us a clear picture of how they work in the chemistry of the body. The smallness of the amount of vitamins that we need daily indicates that they are in some way very different from the rest of our food. Our average daily total food consumption, dry weight, is between a pound and a pound and a half; the quantity of all the vitamins needed totals only 1/300 of an ounce. Consequently, they cannot be needed to replace the gross daily wear and tear on muscles, tissues, etc.

The bulk of our food consists mainly of three classes of substances—proteins, carbohydrates, and fats. Proteins (meat, eggs, cheese, and fish) are required for the construction and repair of muscles and such organs as the liver and kidneys. Carbohydrates (starches and sugars) and fats are sources of energy for the production of work and body heat.

Most of these substances, before they can be used by the body, must first be broken down in the stomach and intestine. This is the process of digestion. The nature of this process is understood immediately if we consider the diet of a baby. This diet is mainly milk. Out of milk the baby builds flesh and bone, blood, hair, skin, and nails, and so on. The way in which this profound transformation occurs is that the materials in the milk are first broken down and then the fragments are rearranged by each tissue according to its special needs. It is the same as if a great brick building were broken down into its constituent bricks. From these bricks it would be possible to build an almost infinite number of different kinds of structures, simply by arranging the bricks differently, into different shapes, different-sized window and door openings, floors, etc. To use the second-hand dealer's phrase, the food is "reconditioned," "rebuilt," in the body, after a preliminary wrecking operation in the gastro-intestinal tract.

The vitamins do not undergo this preliminary disintegration. They are built into the structure of the animal organism as they come. They form parts of the machinery of all the cells of the body. Since the vitamins are continually being worn out and also lost by excretion, the stock must be continually replenished. The vitamins in the food are comparable to the "spare parts" for our cars. Or, to change the figure, the vitamins are the spark in our internal combustion engine. If there are enough vitamins, we have a rich, efficient spark, and the fuel that we take in as food can be efficiently utilized. If the vitamin supply is low, our spark is weak and our fuel is incompletely utilized. The engine loses power, begins to knock, and delivers poor physiological mileage.

Vitamin A, for example, we now know is essential to the mechanism of vision in dim light. A substance in the eye called visual purple is decomposed when light shines in the eye, and re-formed in the dark. The sensation of vision in dim light may be said to be in some way the result of the decomposition of visual purple. In the absence of visual purple an animal is blind in dim light. The return of vision at night after exposure to a glaring light depends on the reconstruction of the visual purple which has been broken down.

The rate at which the visual purple is regenerated is governed by the amount of vitamin A in the diet and hence in the eye. When the amount of this vitamin in the diet is too low, the visual purple is regenerated slowly and imperfectly. The result is that vision in dim light is poor, and becomes progressively worse by exposure to intermittent bright light. If the vitamin A in the diet is increased, the so-called night blindness disappears in a short time, simply because the additional vitamin A enables the chemistry of the eye to utilize the materials necessary for regenerating sufficient visual purple.

So far this discussion, especially in the examples cited, has given special emphasis to the importance of vitamins in preventing or curing various deficiency diseases. But they have an equally important role in maintaining a high general level of health. Literally millions of people who are not actually ill, who do not have definite symptoms of disease, nevertheless suffer continuously from minor aches and pains and discomforts and feel themselves to be below par physically. In the old phrase, they are "enjoying ill health." They are not sick enough to be prevented from following the routine of their daily life and work, but they can do so only at the price of discomfort and disproportionate fatigue. It would be absurd, of course, to indicate vitamins as the cure for all such cases, but for a large class of them vitamins actually do provide the means of bringing them back to par. An instance can be given from the author's own experience.

About six years ago he undertook to obtain an answer to the following question: Is it possible that much of the chronic ill health of middle and old age occurs because the amount of vitamins in the common diet is insufficient for the highest state of health although adequate to prevent serious disease?

There was reason to believe from experimental work on animals that a mild deficiency of vitamin B, for example, may be responsible for much chronic gastro-intestinal distress, lack of energy, recurrent neuritic pains, and so on. This condition is very common. It might pass for a description of average middle age.

This question, of course, had been raised before, but it had not really been settled. Dr. E. D. Kremers and the author undertook to try to obtain a clear answer. Over a period of about four years we collected nearly five hundred such cases of chronic dyspepsia—cases in which dispensaries, sanatoria, and private physicians had been unable to effect any significant or lasting improvement. All that we did, after excluding from the experiment cases of serious organic disease, was to provide a good diet and to enrich it with 750 to 1000 units of vitamin B_1 daily and a corresponding supplement of other members of the B complex.[1] These cases were followed week by week; in many of them we have a daily record extending for as long as four years.

When the results were summarized we found that about 85 per cent of these cases had improved markedly under this very simple regime of enriching the diet with the whole vitamin B complex. Subsequently our findings were completely confirmed by other, independent investigations. We felt justified in concluding, then, that much of the chronic dyspepsia of middle and old age was simply the result of insufficient vitamin B complex in the diet.

Vitamin research is one of the most active fields in chemistry and biology today; we can confidently expect further great extensions of our knowledge of what vitamins are and how they work. But we know enough about them now to be sure that they must be the cornerstone of any sound nutritional scheme. Their detailed place in general diet and the simplest and cheapest ways of securing them will be explained in the ensuing chapters.

---

[1] *The substance originally designated "vitamin B" was later found to consist of several vitamins. Those already identified are B_1 (thiamine), B_2 (flavin or riboflavin; sometimes called vitamin G), nicotinic acid, pantothenic acid, and B_6 (pyridoxin). It is known that there are at least two more members of the B complex, but these have not yet (September 1940) been chemically identified.*

Vitamins and More Abundant Health

ATTEMPTS to change eating habits, like attempts to change any established human practices, are bound to meet vigorous opposition. Frequently such opposition grounds itself on the belief that animals (including human beings) instinctively know what is best for them and that, if left to their own devices, they exercise a wise selection of the foods they need. This doctrine of dietary *laissez-faire* also has a familiar variant: our forefathers, who did not perplex themselves with questions of diet, ate well and achieved mightily; and what was good enough for them ought to be good enough for us. But how well does either square with the facts?

Do We Intuitively Select the Best Food?

This is a common question. It is often followed by the challenge that if the race has managed to survive thus far, there can be little at fault with our diet, so long as we have enough to eat. The following opinion, written by a British medical authority in 1897, represents this point of view:

The generalized food customs of mankind are not to be viewed as random practices adopted to please the palate or gratify an idle or

13

vicious appetite. These customs must be regarded as the outcome of profound instincts which correspond to certain wants of the human economy. They are the fruit of a colossal experience accumulated by countless millions of men through successive generations.

It is true that the "colossal experience accumulated by countless millions of men through successive generations" has enabled the race to survive. But can't we do better than Nature? Scientific research shows that Nature, who is blindly empirical, is not always a reliable guide.

In carefully designed experiments it was found that when an animal had become ill with a severe vitamin deficiency, it selected the proper food *afterward* only if that food gave quick relief and if it had a noticeable smell or color. If the relief was slow, or if the curative substance was incorporated in a food which did not have a distinctive smell or color, the animal did not exercise any "wise" selection.

Food faddists from time to time exhort us to consider the wise Eskimo, who in his native state has never been known to have a decayed tooth. Yet the wise Eskimo is avid for the white man's food when he can get it, although his teeth invariably go to pieces afterward.

It is true that the diet of many native peoples is superior to that of the modern city-dwellers of America and Europe. An American authority, McCollum, has pointed out that the cereal diet with large quantities of leafy vegetables of the peoples of southern and eastern Asia (in former times), and the milk and meat diet of people of more or less arid areas, are both superior to the common diets in America.

But there are native tribes whose diet is worse. Two tribes living in adjacent areas of New Guinea were investigated recently. Both ate far too much starch—much more than we do—and too little protein and fat. Though the condition of the teeth was wretched in both peoples, it was definitely worse in the group whose diet was very low in vitamins A and B. The means of improving the diet is readily available to these people, yet their diet remains poor.

An investigation into the health and diet of another pair of tribes, the Masai and Kikuyu, living side by side in East Africa, was carried out a few years ago. The Masai are a pastoral people whose diet consists almost exclusively of meat, milk, and fresh blood. Their neighbors, the Kikuyu, are agriculturalists. They maintain herds of goats, but these are a form of currency and are rarely used for meat or milk. The diet of the men is almost entirely cereals and potatoes. It is considered effeminate to eat green vegetables; these are eaten only by the women.

The full-grown Masai male is on the average five inches taller and twenty-three pounds heavier than the full-grown Kikuyu male. His muscular strength is nearly twice as great. The Masai boys have only one-fifth the dental defects of the Kikuyu boys. Among the Kikuyu girls (who eat green vegetables) dental defects are only half as frequent as among their brothers.

The Kikuyu are as free and able to choose a good diet as the Masai; yet they fail to do so.

In respect to choosing a good diet it appears that we are all nearly alike, Eskimo, South Sea Islander, African, and American. It was demonstrated more than ten years ago in England and America that the dental health of children can be much improved by certain simple, inexpensive, easy dietary measures. Except in a few free clinics for the poor, and in a few orphan asylums, this work has had practically no influence on the diet of children. Most adults do not obtain enough of the vitamin B complex even when there are no financial reasons for restricting the diet. Expectant and nursing mothers, when they are not especially instructed, fail to drink enough milk. Women are less slow to change their styles, their cosmetics, or the polish of their nails than the family diet.

How Well Did Our Ancestors Feed?

It is often not clear who is meant when we use such terms as "our ancestors," "the race," or "mankind." If we are to consider the diet of our ancestors, we must take into account two kinds of ancestors. The distinction is made by one of the characters in Disraeli's novel *Sybil*, who points out that there are

... *two nations; between whom there is no intercourse and no sympathy; who are as ignorant of each other's habits, thoughts, and feelings as if they were dwellers in different zones, or inhabitants of different planets; who are formed by a different breeding, are fed by a different food, are ordered by different manners, and are not governed by the same laws.* ...
The Rich and the Poor.

The rich, in times past, if we may judge from the records of the English people, ate well. In fact, they overate. Their meals consisted of meat, fish, and fowl, some kind of bread, and enormous quantities of beer and wine. In the time of Henry VIII

The delicate ladies of the court as well as hungry citizens and

robust squires commenced and concluded the day with broiled steaks
or mighty sirloins and flagons of brown ale.[1]

There were practically no vegetables eaten at that time.
The art of what we now call market gardening came into
England from Flanders at about the beginning of the
seventeenth century. A certain Samuel Hartlib, writing in
1655, states that

> *About 50 years ago, about which time* Ingenuities *first began to*
> *flourish in* England; *This* Art *of* Gardening *began to creep into*
> England, *into* Sandwich, *and* Surrey, Fulham, *and other places.*
>
> *Some old men in Surrey, where it flourisheth very much at present,*
> *report, That they knew the first* Gardiners *that came into those*
> *parts, to plant* Cabages, Colleflowers, *and to sow* Turnips,
> Carrets, *and* Parsnips, *to sow* Raith (*or early ripe*) Pease, Rape,
> *all which at that time were great rarities; we having few, or none in*
> England, *but what came from* Holland, *and* Flanders.[2]

But even in 1655, as Hartlib goes on to point out, gardening
was pretty well confined to the area around London. The
"famous Town" of Gravesend, only twenty miles away,
"had not so much as a Mess of Pease, but what came from
London"; and in "divers other places, both in the *North* and
West of *England* . . . the name of *Gardening* and *Howing* is
scarcely known. . . ."

Toward the end of the seventeenth century peas, beans,
cabbages, potatoes, and a few other vegetables were grown.
The potatoes certainly were for human consumption; most
of the other vegetables, it appears, were used mainly for
animal feed.

Samuel Pepys's *Diary* (1660–1669) is a storehouse of

---

[1] *Craik and MacFarlane,* The Pictorial History of England, *1849, vol. II, p. 881.*
[2] Legacie, *p. 9.*

information about one decade of seventeenth-century life, and among other things it gives a good deal of information about the diet of a prosperous Londoner. Pepys was fond of good eating; he records his culinary adventures with gusto. He dines "with a good pig"; he has a "lovely chine of beef," a "good hog's harslet," a "brave plum-porridge"; he gives a dinner which was "noble and enough." But among the numerous items on food and good eating in the *Diary*, vegetables receive only a few mentions. Pepys had carrots as part of an unsatisfactory dinner at his father's house. Twice, in April, asparagus appears in the record. There is one mention of peas, one of radishes. Onions apparently were used for sauce; their single appearance in the *Diary* occurs in connection with the sad case of "W. Boyer, who could not endure onyons in sauce to lamb, but was overcome by the sight of it. . . ." Even more appalling is the only reference to cucumbers: "This day [Sept. 22, 1663] Sir W. Batten tells me that Mr. Newhouse is dead of eating cowcumbers, of which the other day I heard another, I think."

Fruit receives hardly any more attention than vegetables. For one thing, it was dear. In the main, it seems to have been served only on special occasions. There is one mention of melons, one of figs. Strawberries appear more frequently, as June brings them into season. Oranges and lemons were a luxury. Oranges appear most frequently in Pepys's accounts of his visits to the playhouses. There they were sold by the orange women at sixpence apiece (twice the market price). Pepys ruefully notes that on one trip to the theater with his wife and some friends it cost him "8*s*. upon them in oranges."

It is clear from the *Diary* that fruit and vegetables played a negligible part in the diet of Pepys and his prosperous contemporaries. When he and his wife dined alone, their dinner was "good ribs of beef roasted and mince pies," or "a rabbit and two little lobsters," or "a good pie baked of a leg of mutton." For special occasions the menu was more elaborate, but the added dishes were merely more meat or seafood or pastry. The following is a typical example:

We had a fricasee of rabbits and chickens, a leg of mutton boiled, three carps in a dish, a great dish of a side of lamb, a dish of roasted pigeons, a dish of four lobsters, three tarts, a lamprey pie (a most rare pie), a dish of anchovies, good wine of several sorts, and all things mighty noble and to my great content.

The serving of vegetables could not have become general before the nineteenth century. We may deduce this from the records of Arthur Young, who was a student of the condition of agriculture at the end of the eighteenth century. He made a special point of noting, in his wide travels in Great Britain and on the Continent, the prices of human provisions. The following is typical of English prices:

Cheese	3*d.*	*per pound*
Butter	6*d.*	" "
Beef	3½*d.*	" "
Mutton	4*d.*	" "
Veal	3½*d.*	" "
Pork	4*d.*	" "
Bacon	6*d.–*7*d. per pound*	
Milk (an item rarely mentioned)		
	½*d. per pint*	
Potatoes	4*d.–*6*d. per peck*	

The omission of peas, carrots, beans, and cabbages from this list is notable, because Young devoted much space in his journals to the methods used in raising these vegetables, the acreage devoted to them, and lauded and exhorted their use as animal feed, to increase the supply of meat.

The few vegetables that were eaten were cooked, except for radishes and an occasional "sallet." We may be sure that then, even more than now, their vitamins (B_1 and C)—which are lost in injudicious cooking—and their minerals were thrown out in the cooking water.

The English also drank little milk. Young, in a whole volume of his travels in England and Wales, mentions milk only once in his price lists. Probably a little milk was drunk by those who kept cows; the rest was made into cheese and butter, the whey being fed to the hogs. Some cows were kept in the towns; Pepys once mentions seeing a group of milkmaids, their pails garlanded with flowers. But there could have been no very widespread distribution of milk because there was no means of keeping it sweet in transit. As late as 1890, when there had been a definite dairy industry in England for fifteen to twenty years, the per capita daily milk consumption, apart from butter and cheese, was about one-third of a pint; the milk equivalent of the cheese consumed daily in 1890 was another one-third pint per capita.[3]

We may conclude that the diet of the prosperous classes in England until recent times was excessive in calories, protein, and phosphorus; low in calcium and vitamins C and D. The vitamin B content was probably too low for the quantity of food which was consumed. The English showed it in their poor teeth, their gout, and their frequent visits to Bath and the other "waters" to recover from the effects of living too well.

---

[3] *Even now in England there is no improvement in milk consumption. The per capita daily consumption of milk is about two-fifths of a pint; the milk equivalent of cheese, about one-fourth pint. For a good diet today the recommended quantity of milk is one pint per day for an adult, one quart for a child.*

Diet in the United States in earlier times was not much different. For example, in Alice Morse Earle's *The Sabbath in Puritan New England* there is the following description of a supper served on the ordination of a new pastor of the Old South Church in Boston, February 1761:

There were six tables that held one with another eighteen persons each, upon each table a good rich plum pudding, a dish of boil'd pork and fowls, and a corn'd leg of pork with sauce proper for it, a leg of bacon, a piece of alamode beef, a leg of mutton with caper sauce, a roast line of veal, a roast turkey, a venison pastee, besides chess cakes and tarts, cheese and butter . . . they had the best of old cyder, one barrel of Lisbon wine, punch in plenty before and after dinner, made of old Barbados spirit.

Cookery books are another fruitful source of information about the eating habits of our prosperous ancestors. As late as 1882 a leading American expert recommends the following menu[4] for a dinner for twelve people:

Oyster Soup

Smelts à la Tartare

Chicken Vol-au-Vent

Rolled Rib Roast

Polish Sauce   *Grape Jelly*

Cauliflower, with Cream Sauce   *Potato Soufflé*

Rice Croquettes

Larded Grouse with Bread Sauce   *Potatoes à la Parisienne*

Dressed Celery

Royal Diplomatic Pudding

Raspberry Sherbet   *Vanilla Ice Cream*

Cake   *Fruit*

Coffee   *Crackers*   *Cheese*

---

[4] *Maria Parloa,* Miss Parloa's New Cook Book, a Guide to Marketing and Cooking, *Troy, N. Y., 1882, p. 406.*

Nineteenth-century novelists, in England as well as in the United States, set an ample table for their characters. And if one suspects that the testimony of fiction may be somewhat heightened, there is still plenty of evidence of good feeding from other sources. Newspaper accounts of the menus at state dinners and important social functions; diaries, letters, and autobiographies; family records and recollections—all testify to the fact that our well-to-do ancestors provided handsomely for themselves at table. Many middle-aged people still recall nostalgically the plethora of food at old-fashioned country meals. In fact, the tradition is not yet dead of the great family dinner on holidays, birthdays, and other special occasions, with the company spending from one to three hours happily eating themselves into a torpor.

In both England and America our rich and prosperous ancestors fed well. From the point of view of modern dietetics their food was often lacking in many of the elements necessary to maintain a high level of general health, but quantitatively it left nothing to be desired.

Our poor ancestors fared altogether differently. They had a wretched time of it. We read that in Henry VIII's time,

. . . *when the company had finished eating the remaining provisions were sent to the waiters and servants; and when these had sufficiently dined, the fragments were distributed among the poor who waited without the gate.*[5]

The number of poor may be guessed from the figure that "Henry VIII hanged robbers, thieves, and vagabonds no fewer than 72,000."

The following was the menu in an English workhouse (i.e., poorhouse) about 1725:

---

[5] *Craik and MacFarlane,* loc. cit., *vol. II, p. 882.*

. . . *breakfast—bread and cheese four times a week, broth three times a week; dinner—boiled beef and suet pudding three times a week, cold meat three times a week, hasty pudding or milk porridge once a week; supper—bread and cheese or sometimes broth. [On frequent occasions they had beef and pork.] They also had a little garden for herbs, onions, etc.*

We may be pretty sure that the laborer who maintained himself by his own industry could not afford to feed better, and probably not so well as these paupers.[6]

There were workhouses where the diet was better. In one for girls, where the superintendent was especially interested in feeding them well, they had

. . . *beef, pease, potatoes, broth, pease-porridge, milk porridge, bread and cheese, good beer (such as we drink at our own tables), cabbage, carrots, turnips, etc., in which we took the advice of our physician, and bought the best of every sort.*[7]

This was a remarkably wise physician for those days.

Then, as now, there were complaints that the poor were too well kept by the parish to accept work when it was offered them.

In his travels in Wales in 1776 Young found that the food of the poor was bread and cheese, some milk, "no meat, except on Sunday." In one locality, whose diet in the light of our modern knowledge was rather better than elsewhere, he found that

The poor live on barley-bread, cheese, and butter; not one in ten have either cows or pigs, fare very poorly and rarely touch meat. Their

---

[6] *Craik and MacFarlane, loc. cit., vol. IV, p. 846.*
[7] *Idem.*

little gardens they plant with cabbages, carrots, leeks, and potatoes.[8]

These people fared moderately well in summer, except that they ate too little animal protein. In winter they must have fared poorly indeed.

We may obtain a further idea of the state of the poor from the budget which Young computed for a family in Northamptonshire in 1790. This family consisted of a farm laborer, his wife, and five children, the eldest sixteen years of age. The wife and the four youngest children were lace workers. The combined family earnings were £35 2s. per year. Their weekly expenditures for food were itemized as follows:

Bread	6s. 6d.
[apparently home-baked, half of barley, half of wheat, presumably the whole grains]	
Salt	½d.
Bacon *[2 lbs. per week]*	1s. 4d.
Tea, sugar, and butter	2½d.
[certainly less than ½ lb. weekly]	
Cheese, ½ lb.	2½d.
Beer	6d.

Apropos of this family Young comments approvingly:

The state of the poor in general, in this country is advantageous, owing very much to lace making. The wives and children are all employed in lace making; they begin at six and seven years old. . . . It is a great object to all the poor; the trade is now very brisk, and the dealers have made much money for four or five years past.

How was it possible to bring up children on this diet? The

---

[8] Arthur *Young*, Tours in England and Wales. (*No. 14 in Series of Reprints of Scarce Tracts in Economics and Political Science, the London School of Economics and Political Science*), *p. 9*.

man, judging from his wages, obtained a good deal of meat for about nine weeks during harvest and haying time, and plenty of beer at all times, from his employers. The family had no cow; they must have been given some milk, which they put in their tea. Certainly it was the very large amount of whole-grain bread they ate, apparently more than two pounds daily per capita, which saved them. This gave them daily per capita nearly 1000 International Units of vitamin B_1, which is above the requirement for excellent health.

Their diet as given indicates that their crude home-made beer, which gave them some protein, was practically their only source of vitamin C, and hence their only protection against scurvy. They must have been given a few potatoes, and possibly they stole, found, or were given some apples occasionally. These incidental items could not have been large, or Young would have noted them.

This diet as it stands was low in protein, calcium, and vitamins A and C. The children, working the long hours they did, could have got very little exposure to sunshine, which would have been their principal source of vitamin D. Yet this diet was not very different from that of the poorest 10 per cent of the British people today, except that it was far superior in vitamin B, thanks to their whole-grain bread.

What the People of Iowa Ate

About the turn of the century a study was made of the diet of the people of Iowa. On the basis of data collected in this study,[9] plus our present knowledge of nutritional require-

---

[9] Fred Clark, "*What the People of Iowa Eat*," Medical News, *vol. LXXIII (Aug. 1898), p, 193.*

ments, we can see how adequate their diet was. In the following condensation, the daily intake of the most necessary nutritional elements is given for an unskilled laborer, a farmer, and a banker. These are chosen as representing three different economic levels and thus giving a fair cross-section of the population. The figures in bold-face type call attention to inadequate amounts of the respective elements.

	Calories	Protein	Calcium	Vitamin A	Vitamin B_1	Vitamin C
		Grams	Milli-grams	Inter-national Units	Inter-national Units	Milli-grams
Unskilled laborer	3000	83	**347**	**2700**	**403**	**10**
Farmer	3500	62	**388**	6400	500	124
Banker	3400	136	**434**	6100	**272**	77
Standard adequate diet—U. S. Dept. of Agriculture	3000 to 3500	67	680	6000	500	75

Clark may have underestimated somewhat the milk, fruit, and leafy vegetables eaten. But even when generous allowance is made for this possible underestimate, all the diets were deficient in calcium; two were deficient in vitamin B_1 and one was deficient in vitamin C. In general, all the diets were short of the amounts necessary for good health. Consequently, Clark's comment on the health of Iowans on this diet is not surprising:

The bulk of the country doctor's practice in this part of Iowa . . . consists of constipation, the dyspepsias, chronic rheumatisms and myalgias, acne, eczema and their results. Constipation with the women is universal, and is common with the men. In the summer this is somewhat lessened by the free use of vegetables and uncooked fruits. Dyspepsia—chronic gastric catarrh—with its results is, in Jefferson county, one of the most prevalent diseases the doctor is called on to treat.

Diet and Health

The ill-chosen or inadequate nourishment of rich and poor must have been one of the factors responsible for the high mortality rates in times past. Today the number of deaths per 1000 of population between the ages of fifteen and forty-five in England and Scotland is about one-half what it was a hundred years ago. The expectation of life is double what it was. Of course, a number of factors contributed to the great improvement in health during the last century, notably the new knowledge and the resulting better control of infectious diseases. Improved nutrition doubtless contributed also.

We may guess this from some facts that bear indirectly on this question. Children all over the world, in Europe, America, and parts of Asia, have increased in height and weight in the past thirty years when compared with older generations. But in some groups there has been little or no change.

The children of the English working class today are no taller or heavier than children of the same class were in 1879. The Chinese children in San Francisco today after the age of nine do not reach present-day standards in Canton, the province from which most of the Chinese of San Francisco come, and are far behind the Cantonese children of Hawaii.

The Japanese children on the Pacific Coast of the United States, born in America of Japanese parents, are 7 per cent taller than Japanese children in Japan today, 20 per cent heavier, their legs are 9 per cent longer, and their chest circumference is 7 per cent greater. In fact, Japanese children in the Los Angeles region today are, until the age of sixteen, taller and heavier than the children of the English working class. An English working man (employed), aged twenty, is on the average only about one inch taller than a Japanese of the same age born of Japanese parents on the Pacific Coast of the United States. At the age of eighteen the English working man is about six inches shorter than a boy of the same age of the English upper classes.

The inferior height and weight of the working-class children in England and the Chinese children in San Francisco, as compared to the Japanese children on the American West Coast, are in all probability due to differences in the whole set of circumstances which usually go together—nutrition, housing, and hygiene. The diet and the whole mode of life of the Chinese in San Francisco are like those of the poor in the Chinese cities; the diet of the Japanese in that city is better, though still not up to a wholly desirable standard.

In studies of the diet of families in Pasadena (near Los Angeles) it was found that even the poor obtained fair amounts of vitamin A and an abundance of vitamin C. Fresh green vegetables are cheap all the year around and are bought by the poor. On the other hand, Orr's estimates of the diet of the British people[10] indicate that the lower half of the population of England and Scotland (graduated on the basis of income) are subsisting on inadequate amounts of vitamins A and C; 30 per cent are obtaining an inadequate total number of calories and insufficient calcium, phosphorus, and iron; and 10 per cent, too little protein. An additional contributory factor on the American West Coast is the larger number of hours of sunshine per year than in England. This increases the amount of vitamin D.[11]

---

[10] *John Boyd Orr*, Food, Health and Income, *London, 1936.*
[11] *For a full discussion of vitamin D and sunshine see Chapter VII.*

These considerations suggest the great increase which can
be effected in the stature and general health of a whole population by improvement in diet. It would be extremely interesting if adequate data could be collected on the amount of
chronic ill health in adults in Europe and America fifty and
a hundred years ago and today. To what extent are differences in nutrition responsible for the difference in the fashion
of female beauty then and now? The English Pre-Raphaelite
painters depicted a tall woman with a swelling at the base of
the neck, pale and "delicate." The swelling of the neck was
the result of dietary deficiency of iodine; the paleness and
"delicacy" were the anemia of chlorosis—the result of a deficiency of iron. Compare her with the girl on the American
magazine covers today!

It is difficult, if not invidious, to determine which is most
important: the abolition of slums, better sanitation and hygiene, or a better diet. The advantages that result from improvement in one are limited by inadequacies in the others.
Social reform campaigns should attempt to improve all three
together. On the other hand, it may be easier to improve
the national diet first. Such an improvement calls for no
large expenditure of public money.

The synthesis of vitamins on a commercial scale and the
manufacture of vitamin concentrates have now reached a
stage which would make it possible to add vitamins to foods
during and after processing. For instance, the vitamin B complex could be added to white flour and white sugar at the
mills and refineries; vitamins A and the B complex to canned
goods at the canneries; and vitamin C to soft drinks at the
bottling works. Thus everyone, rich and poor alike, would
be assured of a vitamin intake adequate by the highest nutritional standards. This need not affect the taste of the foods;

it would not interfere with industrial processing; and the added cost to the consumer need be only negligible.

The Next Great Public Health Undertaking

The next great public health undertaking will be an attack on chronic ill health, the result of poor nutrition. The whole problem, from the viewpoint of tactics, can be stated in terms of providing enough vitamins. If enough of these are provided from natural sources, all the other elements necessary to a good diet will be provided automatically.

One of the obstacles in educating the public to a richer vitamin diet is the opinion held in some medical circles that any mixed diet contains an adequate supply of vitamins. This opinion is correct or incorrect according to what is meant by "adequate."

The early work on vitamins emphasized how small the necessary amounts of vitamins are, when those amounts are expressed in pounds or ounces. It was also found that nearly all animal and plant tissues contain some vitamins; otherwise, they could not have lived. And so it was concluded that we in the United States obtain enough of the vitamins.

"Enough" for what? Enough to prevent severe deficiency diseases such as xerophthalmia and beri-beri? Yes. Enough to prevent rickets and poor dental health? No. To prevent defective vision in dim light in at least 5 to 10 per cent of the population? No. To prevent constipation and gastro-intestinal ill health in an even larger percentage of adults? No.

The fact is that it is nearly impossible to obtain enough of all the vitamins for the highest state of health from the ordinary American diet, and the American urban diet is better than that in Europe. The modern tendency toward dietary fads, reducing diets, and such refinements as white flour has aggravated the situation.

It has been found in the last few years that there are degrees of vitamin deficiency. Between a condition of severe deficiency such as exists in beri-beri or scurvy, for instance, and a high state of health (as far as nutrition is concerned) there is a range of intermediate states. For example, about 250 units of vitamin B_1 daily will prevent beri-beri; but 750 to 1000 units are commonly required for really good health. In other words, excellent health is more than the absence of outright disease.

The following experiment will demonstrate this point. Two large groups of rats were kept on an identical diet, except that in one lot the vitamin B intake was kept at such a level that the rate of growth was only slightly subnormal. In the other lot the vitamin B intake provided for normal growth. The first group reached adult size only slightly later than the normal group. In the subnormal Group I, 38 per cent survived after two years; in the normal Group II, 64 per cent. In Group I, 33 per cent had gastric ulcers; in Group II, 2 per cent. In Group I, there were 14 pregnancies with 78 young born; in Group II, 94 pregnancies with 635 young. In Group I, 16 per cent of the young survived one month; in Group II, 88 per cent.

This experiment showed that a small deficiency in vitamin B, which was barely perceptible in the growth rate of the rat, had disastrous consequences during a period which would correspond to middle age in a human being. The shorter life of the rat permits us to see more clearly—because it happens more quickly—what is going on in us at a much slower rate.

An objection may be made that in this experiment one group of rats was maintained on a diet which was actually deficient in vitamin B. This experiment, it might be said, affords no argument in favor of increasing the vitamin B intake over that required for a normal rate of growth. The objection was answered in the following experiment. Rats were fed a diet consisting essentially of one part of dried whole milk and five parts of ground whole wheat. These animals were normal in every respect—rate of growth, duration of reproductive period, and length of life. The diet was certainly adequate. Another group of the same rats was fed one part dried whole milk and two parts ground whole wheat. There was therefore twice as much milk in this diet. This second group of rats surpassed the others in rate of growth, duration of the reproductive period, and length of life. Subsequent experiments showed that the increased length of life cannot be attributed to any one factor in the milk, but to a combination of the factors there: the calcium, the vitamin B_2, and possibly still other factors.

Where to Begin?

Of course the place to begin is with the children. Analysis of the mortality statistics in England, Scotland, and Sweden for the past hundred and fifty years showed that the mortality rate of any generation from the time it is fifteen years of age until it is seventy-five is fixed by the environmental conditions during the first fifteen years of life. Any improvement attained in environmental, social, and nutritional conditions in any era is reflected in improved adult health and increased length of life of those who were children in this period. In the words of one group of investigators

> . . . *care of the children during the first 10–15 years of life is of supreme importance. It is at this period of life that improved environment exercises its effect most promptly and furthermore the improved physique built up during this period would seem to be of decisive effect at all later ages.*[12]

This conclusion is confirmed by experiments on the growth of animals. To attain maximum, even normal size, a normal growth rate must be maintained in the young. If there is any prolonged retardation of growth in early life it is not fully made up later.

Quality vs. Quantity

Some of the latest studies on dietary factors affecting growth have brought out the exceedingly interesting and important point of how much more important quality is than quantity. When rats were given a diet adequate in minerals, vitamins, and first-class (animal) protein but so deficient in calories that the growth rate was retarded, the adult size attained was of course subnormal, yet the health of the adult and the length of life were normal, even though the amount of calories was subnormal during most of the life of the animal. In fact, the males in the retarded group lived somewhat longer; there was no difference in the females.

It must be emphasized that the diet in this experiment was rich in minerals, vitamins, and animal protein. The only real

[12] *W. O. Kermack, A. G. McKendrick, and P. L. Finlay,* Lancet, *vol. I (1934), p. 698.*

dietary restriction was in the number of calories (i.e., the *amount* of food) consumed. In all experiments where the quality of the diet was improved by enriching it with minerals, vitamins, and animal protein the results were increased stature, increased length of life, a longer period of vigorous adult life, and better adult health.

It is a conclusion of the greatest importance for those engaged in providing relief for large populations that in the long view the quality of the diet is more important than the quantity. Where funds for food are limited and some compromise must be made, it is wiser to stint on the quantity in order to enrich the quality as much as possible. Animals and babies on vitamin-deficient diets may die with full stomachs.

In Spain as a result of the civil war there was an appalling infant mortality. In November 1938, there were 40,000 cases of the vitamin-deficiency diseases pellagra and beri-beri in Madrid alone. This was much more the result of malnutrition than of undernutrition. Toward the end of the civil war the safe arrival of a food ship from the United States in one of the Loyalist ports received wide notice. Yet the amount of food carried was only enough for Barcelona for one day. The same amount of money and cargo space would have carried more than enough vitamins and vitamin concentrates to cure the deficiency diseases which had already appeared and to safeguard for many months against their wider occurrence.

The brewer's yeast thrown away as refuse by the breweries of France and Belgium could have been had for the small cost of drying and hauling. This alone would have prevented the pellagra and beri-beri, and it would have insured a health level higher than in pre-civil war Spain.

We have heard many reports recently that the emergency rations of German parachute troops and motorized divisions are highly fortified with vitamins. Stories of the same sort have also been circulated about the rations of munitions workers. If these reports are true, they provide an apt illustration of emphasis on the quality of diet. For the general population of Germany, however, the situation would appear to be quite different. Reliable data on the general diet are not available, but from *The Nazi Primer* we can get a good idea of what conditions are like for the majority of people.

The Nazi Primer is designed to instruct German school children in the fundamental doctrines of National Socialism and to regiment them in carrying out those doctrines. One section details the dietary measures which must be followed as a patriotic obligation, in order to make Germany as independent as possible of imported foodstuffs.

From the economic point of view, the *Primer* urges,[13] it is desirable to have:

A Greater Use of	*The Same Use of*	*Less Use of*
potatoes	bread, bakery products	beef
sugar, marmalade	flour	veal
skimmed milk	pork	butter
curds	wild game	grease
hulled barley, grits	fowl	bacon
oatmeal	eggs	margarine
sago	rice	vegetable oils, fat
artificial honey	cocoa	buckwheat
buttermilk	fruit	millet
Hartz and Limburger cheese	peas, beans	imported vegetables, especially im-
native vegetables	lentils	ported early vege-
fish	whole milk	tables
mutton	dried fruits	whole cheese
rabbit meat	honey	

This patriotic diet provides no improvement in vitamin B, which is already insufficient; no improvement in vitamin C;

---

[13] Handbuch für die Schulungsarbeit in der HJ. vom deutschen Volk und seinem Lebensraum, *Munich, 1937. Translated as* The Nazi Primer, *by Harwood L. Childs, New York, 1938, p. 233.*

and a definite deficiency in vitamin A. If continued for any length of time it will inevitably result in a lowering of the general level of health and is very likely to produce vitamin-deficiency disease.

If a large part of Continental Europe should suffer from a serious food shortage, if not actual famine, any relief agencies—whether national or international—that attempt to deal with the situation must choose between trying to maintain the quantity or the quality of the diet. Certainly the choice should be quality, and quality means first of all an adequate intake of vitamins. Maintaining quality can be accomplished more economically, especially where large numbers of people are involved; it produces better results as far as general health is concerned; and, most important, it safeguards children against the disastrous results that come from vitamin deficiency during their critical first ten or fifteen years.

Vitamins Are Not Cure-Alls

Of course vitamins are not cure-alls. For example, they do not afford increased protection against serious infections such as pneumonia, whooping cough, measles, or influenza. They do not hasten recovery from infectious diseases, even when administered in large doses. They will neither prevent nor cure most cases of heart disease. They will not cure pyorrhea in adults. They will not do much even for colds.

But when vitamins are used extensively and intelligently, as they can be with little difficulty, what is now a fair average state of health will be thought rather poor health. The "average adult" will less frequently be conscious of his insides, his teeth, joints, and nerves. He will begin to feel and be old at a later age. All that this calls for is the use of the knowledge we already have.

The proper place for this knowledge is in the cookery books rather than on a shelf in the physicians' offices. The prevention of serious diseases is only the second-best use of vitamins; their best use is to promote the highest state of health. This will be attained when vitamin lore is domesticated in the kitchen. A good working knowledge of vitamins should be part of the education of every girl.

CHAPTER III

Vitamin Units

Why They Must Be Measured and How

TO PROCEED about the business of obtaining an adequate supply of vitamins in our food we should ask and be able to answer such questions as these: How many units of each of the vitamins do I need? Approximately how many units of each of the vitamins are there in my present diet? What is the cheapest or the best way of securing the vitamins which my family and I require?

The trouble here is that accurate information is quantitative information; that is, it is a matter of detailed arithmetic. Chapter X and the tables on pages 167 to 193 will, the author hopes, help the reader over this difficulty.

In order to determine how much of any one vitamin there is in any given food, extracting the vitamin and weighing it are out of the question. The quantity involved is much too small. For instance, the amount of vitamin B_1 in a cupful of whole wheat is about one-millionth of an ounce. And the labor of extraction and isolation would be enormous.

There are easier methods which are as good or better. These fall into two main classes: biological, and chemical or physical. In biological methods of assay a group of young animals is used. Animals are good experimental material because their physiological reactions are sufficiently similar to those of human beings and their shorter life-span enables us to see in them in a brief space of time what is going on in us at a much slower rate. The animals are fed a diet adequate in every respect except that the one vitamin under consideration is rigorously excluded. After some time on this deficient diet the animals stop growing or the characteristic deficiency disease appears. The minimum amount of a foodstuff which will restore a normal rate of growth or cure the disease is then designated as one unit of the particular vitamin which was missing from the diet.[1]

The chemical and physical methods of assaying vitamins come later, after a good deal has been learned of their chemistry, and the actual chemical or physical method used is different for each vitamin. These methods are quicker and less expensive than the biological methods, but from time to time they must be checked by biological assays. Where there is disagreement between results obtained by the two methods, the biological values are preferred.

The determination of the human requirement of the different vitamins constitutes a whole series of separate problems. For instance, it does not follow that because a human adult weighs three hundred times as much as a rat he will require three hundred times as much vitamin A. He may require more or less. The requirement of that or of any other vitamin will depend on his physiological condition, the climate he lives in, the amount of physical work he is doing, and so on. There is a greater requirement of all the vitamins during pregnancy and lactation. It is possible that adults may not require any more vitamin D than children do, if they require any at all. To determine human requirements,

---

[1] *Different vitamins require different test animals; the rat or the pigeon is used for vitamin B assays; the guinea pig for vitamin C; the rat for vitamin D. The selected test animals are standardized with respect to their age, weight, previous diet, and, sometimes, the diet of their parents.*

the findings in animal tests provide indispensable guides. But the final decision regarding human requirements must rest on findings made on human beings. And we must distinguish also between the minimum requirement for the prevention of manifest disease and the amount which will insure the highest state of health.

The foodstuffs are, of course, the natural sources of the vitamins. But under certain circumstances—as will appear in the following chapters—it is desirable to obtain a richer supply. This is available in two forms: synthetic vitamins and vitamin concentrates. The synthetic vitamins are those which investigators have learned to produce artificially (that is, to synthesize) after discovering the chemical structure of the original vitamin. For ordinary purposes the synthetic vitamins are added to some neutral substance, because if they were undiluted the amount involved in a dose would be so small that measuring it out would be practically impossible. For example, the pure vitamin D (ergosterol irradiated with ultraviolet light) is added to corn oil. The resulting combination is known commercially as viosterol, the dosage of which is measured by the drop.

Vitamin concentrates are obtained by first finding a rich natural source of the desired vitamin and then refining it so that the vitamin is left in a much more highly concentrated form than it can ever be found in nature. One of the commercial preparations of the vitamin B complex provides a good illustration. The rich natural source in this case is rice bran. The vitamin B is dissolved out of the bran by a suitable solvent. Then the solvent is got rid of; and the final product —a thick, sirupy substance—while not the pure vitamin B complex, is so rich in it that one tablespoonful daily provides an abundant amount of the complex for a grown person.

In discussions of the vitamin content of foods or in advertisements or labels of commercially synthesized or concentrated vitamin products, the reader may be troubled by what
seems to be a bewildering variety of measurement systems. He
may encounter measurement by units, e.g., Sherman Units,
Sherman-Bourquin Units, International Units; and measurement by weight in grams, milligrams, or gammas (a gamma
—γ—is 1/1000 of a milligram). Measurement by units is the
result of biological assays, and the common practice is to
name the unit after the investigator who made the assays.
International Units represent an attempt to bring the unit
measurements into a single, internationally accepted system.

Measurement by weight comes after the chemical structure
of the vitamin has been determined and it has been synthesized. So for most of the vitamins the progression is from
biological assays and measurement by units to analysis and
synthesis and measurement by weight. Research is proceed-
ing so vigorously now that we can anticipate a rather rapid
transference to the weight system.

All this may seem to explain the situation without offering
the layman any very helpful means of finding his way through
its complexities. But the difficulty disappears if we remember
the following: for ordinary nutritional purposes—that is, for
making sure that our daily diet contains the desired amount
of vitamins—we need to know only two things: (1) the daily
human requirement of the vitamin involved, and (2) the
amount of the various vitamins in the foods which will make
up our bill of fare. As long as these two things are expressed in
the same system of measurement, it makes no difference what
system is used. In the tables on pages 167 to 171 the reader
will find this information in convenient form for daily use.

CHAPTER IV

Vitamin A

THE attention we need pay the amount of vitamin A in the diet varies with geography. In the United States and Canada, fortunately, there is practically no grave vitamin A deficiency. In southern Mexico, on the other hand, one in five of the children of the poor suffers from xerophthalmia, a disease which is the result of severe vitamin A deficiency, and which, if unchecked, leads to blindness and early death from pneumonia.

Signs of Severe Vitamin A Deficiency

The first visible signs of vitamin A deficiency in human beings are dryness of the skin and eruptions where hairs come through the skin. These may occur on any part of the body except the face. In babies the deficiency may show itself as an increased susceptibility to eczema and napkin rash.

In severe deficiency the characteristic disturbances appear in the lining membranes of the eyes, bronchial tubes, intestinal, urinary, and reproductive tracts. These structures contain glandular elements the secretions of which become defective and scanty; as a consequence the membrane linings are unable to resist the invasion of bacteria which normally are harmless. The common result in the young is a severe infection of the eyelids and eyeball (xerophthalmia) in which the whole eyeball runs with pus. These children are abnormally susceptible also to severe respiratory infections. In adults there are gastrointestinal disturbances, and sterility because of failure of the glandular elements of the reproductive apparatus.

Vitamin A deficiency runs parallel with a dietary deficiency of animal fats (except lard).

Mild Vitamin A Deficiency

While there is little serious vitamin A deficiency in the United States, there is fairly widespread mild deficiency. Some observers assert that as many as 50 per cent of normal children and adults are mildly deficient in vitamin A. The most conservative figures, obtained by careful laboratory methods, indicate that at least 5 per cent of ordinary medical patients are deficient.

The signs of vitamin A deficiency in children are retarded growth, a somewhat greater susceptibility to infections, and impairment of the healthy development of teeth and bones. Their life-span is also likely to be shorter than it otherwise might have been. It is not known at present how late in childhood this harm can be completely repaired. Once the deficiency is detected, the child should be given more than the normally adequate amount of vitamin A for at least a year.

In adults, the commonest sign of mild vitamin A deficiency is glare blindness and subnormal vision in dim light.

It is so easy to obtain an adequate amount of vitamin A in the diet that any deficiency, no matter in how small a proportion of the population, is completely unnecessary.

Difficulty in Night Driving a Mild Vitamin A Deficiency

A young man of thirty-one was out driving his car one evening when he heard the familiar and ominous "Pull over to the side of the road." The police officer who stopped him threatened him with arrest for drunken driving, pointing out that he had been driving on the wrong side of the road. The young man had not been drinking, but neither had he been aware that he was driving on the wrong side of the road.

He confessed that driving an automobile at night was difficult, especially when trying to pass an oncoming car. Even dim headlights dazzled him. Under such circumstances he drove, as he put it, "entirely by instinct."

Five years before, fearing a gain in weight, he had cut out of his diet all dairy products and many vegetables. Following this, his skin gradually grew dry and began to itch. His hair became dry and brittle and lusterless and fell out in increasing amounts. When he went into a darkened motion-picture theater, he had to be guided by his wife, and the pictures seemed blurred for five or ten minutes.

Medical examination after this difficulty with the policeman disclosed, in addition, inflammation and dryness of the outer eyeball, and that he was unable to see a luminous watch-dial in the dark.

His case was intermediate between mild and severe vitamin A deficiency, brought on because his restricted diet had eliminated most of the natural sources of vitamin A. His defective vision and the diseased condition of his skin, hair, and eyes, were cured in three weeks by the addition to his diet of butter, milk, carrots, and 30,000 units of vitamin A daily.

A person with mild deficiency may be unaware of his defective vision in dim light. Thus there are reports of two chauffeurs who had had six accidents, with loss of life. They were tested and found to be skillful and careful drivers. But someone pointed out that all the accidents had occurred at night, whereas the driving tests had been made during the day. The two men were then examined for their ability to see in dim light, and both were found to be markedly subnormal. They were suffering from vitamin A deficiency, mild enough so that they were unaware of it, but certainly serious in its consequences.

Since then it has been reported that from 5 to 10 per cent of all automobile drivers have difficulty in seeing at night or complain of glare blindness.[1]

Human Requirements of Vitamin A

A growing child requires 3000 International Units of vitamin A daily; an adult, 6000 to 8000 daily.

This estimate, and those for the other vitamins in the succeeding chapters, are several times the amounts necessary to prevent acute deficiency disease. They are estimates of the requirements for the best state of health.

Babies and Vitamin A

A child is born with a low vitamin A reserve. The mother's milk is not rich enough to build up this reserve quickly, even

---

[1] *The rate of recovery from momentary glare blindness is now the basis of a number of clinical methods used for estimating the amount of vitamin A actually in the body.*

when the mother's diet is enriched with vitamin A concentrates. Babies should therefore be given a vitamin A supplement, from 1000 to 3000 units daily, as soon as possible. If the baby is bottle-fed and dried milk is the chief source of its milk, this supplement is an urgent necessity because of the loss of the vitamin A in the storage of dried milk. The amount of vitamin A in the diet of the young exercises an important influence on their health in later life.

The nursing mother requires more than the normally adequate amount of this vitamin. Ten thousand units a day arc not excessive for her.

Vitamin A in Foods

In assessing the relative values of different foodstuffs as sources of Vitamin A (and of other vitamins) in human dietaries, it must be borne in mind that the real dietetic value of any particular foodstuff depends not only upon its vitamin A content calculated on a weight basis, but also upon the amount which with convenience may be included in a normal diet. Thus milk and butter, while being relatively poor in vitamin A compared on a weight basis with cod-liver oil, are nevertheless extremely valuable sources of this factor, owing to the prominent position which they occupy in the normal human diet.[2]

Vitamin A is soluble in fats; it is insoluble in water. This is the reason that all of the vitamin A in milk is in the cream; in the egg, in the yolk. When the diet is low in suitable fats and in green leafy vegetables—the meaning of "suitable" will be brought out shortly—there is danger of vitamin A deficiency. In Denmark during the war of 1914–1918, nearly

---

[2] *British Medical Research Council report on vitamins.*

all the butter was exported because of the high prices of dairy products in the belligerent countries, and margarine, which contains no vitamin A, was substituted for it. Soon a number of children were stricken with xerophthalmia. It became necessary for the Danish government to limit the quantity of butter which could be exported. The xerophthalmia then practically disappeared.

In vegetables vitamin A is present not as such but in the form of four members of a group of bright yellow substances called carotenoids. These four are converted in the animal (in the liver, probably) into vitamin A. (Vitamin A itself is a very pale yellow.) For this reason, in selecting vegetable sources of vitamin A, it is a fairly safe guide, when there are two forms of a vegetable, one yellow or green and the other white, to choose the yellow or green. The yellow variety contains carotenoids and is therefore a source of vitamin A, whereas the white variety contains none. Some examples of this difference are yellow and white potatoes, the outer green leaves of lettuce and the inner white ones, green and bleached asparagus and celery.

In milk (cream and butter) and eggs the vitamin A is partly vitamin A and partly carotenoids. The proportions vary according to the state and nutrition of the cows and hens. For nearly all nutritional purposes the relative amount of each is immaterial.

It is a pity that parsley is used mainly for decoration, for it is a very rich vegetable source of vitamin A. One-third ounce (fresh weight) daily will supply one-third the total requirement of an adult. This one item of quantitative scientific information, if practically applied, might go a long way toward remedying the situation in regions where there is a wide-spread vitamin A deficiency.

Another excellent source of vitamin A is dandelion leaves. They contain per ounce about 6000 units of potential vitamin A (carotenoids), which is a day's requirement for an adult. A friend of the author's recalls that in the Middle West thirty years ago dandelion greens were a common substitute for spinach at country dinners. Their reappearance on the bill of fare should be encouraged, either cooked like spinach or, better still, served as salad greens. Perhaps we can dig dandelions out of our lawns with more enthusiasm if we know that we are salvaging one of the best sources of vitamin A.

The next-best vegetable sources are, in the order of their richness, chard, chicory, turnip greens, spinach, watercress, kale, sweet potatoes, and carrots. These vegetables, plus tomatoes and dairy products, are the main sources of vitamin A in the ordinary diet.

Curiously, apricots are richer in vitamin A than any other fruit. One large apricot contains one-sixth of the entire requirement of an adult for a day.

For practical purposes vitamin A may be considered as absent from white beans, beets, cauliflower, cucumbers, white potatoes, turnips, white onions, unpolished rice, apples, orange and pineapple juice, grapes, and watermelons. There is only a negligible amount of vitamin A in bread.

Is Vegetable Vitamin A (Carotenoids) Used by Human Beings?

Some observations have been reported recently to the effect that the carotenoids in spinach and carrots are not utilized by human beings. If this is true, these, among the richest vegetable sources of vitamin A, are useless in the human diet for this purpose. But it is improbable that these observations are entirely correct. There is no question that the most potent of the carotenoids, beta carotene, passes through the intestinal wall into the body of the rat, the usual test animal for vitamin A. The figures for the vitamin A contents of vegetables were obtained by feeding them to the rat. Nevertheless, the observations above are a warning that it is inadvisable to rely exclusively on vegetables for vitamin A. The dairy products, milk, cream, butter, and eggs, are thoroughly safe sources of vitamin A for human nutrition.

There are other reasons, in this same connection, for the inclusion of fats in the human diet. Fats (and bile) are necessary for the absorption of beta carotene from the intestine even in animals; and fat in the diet tends to prevent the vitamin A reserves in the liver from too rapid depletion, that is, from being wasted. Lard and vegetable fats and oils that contain no vitamin A serve equally well for this purpose.

Mineral oil, however, retards and in large doses will stop completely the absorption of vitamin A or carotenoids from the intestine. This is one of several reasons against the habitual use of mineral oil as a laxative.

Margarine

The oils of such seeds as cottonseed, linseed, and sesame, of olives and soy beans, contain no significant amounts of vitamin A. Margarine which is made of vegetable fats therefore contains no vitamin A unless it is added.

Recently vitamins A and D have been incorporated into some brands of commercial margarine. One variety has about half the vitamin A content of a good grade of butter. This practice deserves encouragement because margarine has approximately the same caloric value as butter, and it is cheaper. If enough vitamin A could be added to margarine with little additional cost, it would provide an adequate substitute to those unable to afford butter.

The purchaser must be on his guard here. If the price of the margarine is higher because it contains vitamin A, he should compute how many vitamin units he will obtain for the additional price and compare this additional cost with what he can buy in the form of concentrates of the fish-liver oils. No brand of margarine should be purchased for its vitamin A content unless the number of units per pound is stated plainly on the wrapper.

The *Journal of the American Medical Association* (August 12, 1939, p. 594) calls attention to an anomalous situation. The Bureau of Animal Industry of the Department of Agriculture, which has jurisdiction over oleomargarines made from animal fat, has ruled that vitamins come under the head of "possibly harmful and deleterious substances" and hence may not be added to these oleomargarines. But margarines made from vegetable fats and oils come under the jurisdiction of a different bureau, which permits the addition of small quantities of fish-liver oils. In some European countries no margarine may be sold unless it is fortified with vitamins A and D.

Animal Sources of Vitamin A

About 90 per cent of the vitamin A in an animal is in the liver. There is very little in the muscle (flesh). For example, canned salmon is sometimes advertised as containing vitamin A, but the number of units is not given. It is true that salmon flesh does contain more vitamin A than does the flesh of most other fish. Nevertheless, it does not contain enough to be considered a significant source of vitamin A in the usual human diet.

Lard contains no vitamin A.

Vitamin A Concentrates

The richest sources of vitamin A are the fish-liver oils, especially halibut, cod, and turbot. Halibut-liver oil contains approximately a hundred times as much as cod-liver oil. These oils are now sold with a standardized and specified vitamin A and D content. Their relative value should be estimated strictly on the basis of the number of units of the desired vitamin at the price.

Losses in Cooking, Canning, and Storage

The important point to be borne in mind regarding vitamin A in cooking, canning, and storage is that the vitamin is lost if fats become rancid or are heated in the presence of air. In the absence of air (oxygen) there is no loss, even though they may become rancid. But rancidity usually occurs in the presence of air.

None of the vitamin A in milk is lost in pasteurization, or in canning. When boiling milk it is better to bring the milk quickly to the boil than to keep it warm in an open pot. Powdered whole milk loses about 60 per cent of its vitamin A content on storage for nine months.

Butter loses little vitamin A on storage if it is stored in airtight containers. Some of the vitamin A content is lost when butter is cooked; it is entirely destroyed in frying.

Dried fruits and vegetables lose one-half or more of their vitamin A content in the process of drying.

Does Vitamin A Prevent Infection?

Vitamin A has been called the "anti-infective vitamin." This name implies that by the consumption of large doses of vitamin A one acquires an increased ability to resist infection. This would be welcome news if it were true, but a number of careful investigations have shown that it is not true. No close correlation could be found between unsatisfactory diet and the occurrence of bronchitis, in the incidence of and recovery from pneumonia, or in the complications following scarlet fever. There may be some slight value in taking large doses of vitamin A as protection against colds, but the beneficial results even here are at best discernible only in extensive statistical surveys. The appellation "anti-infective vitamin" should therefore be discouraged. It is certainly an overstatement. It might lead people to take undue risks in exposure to colds or more serious infections in the mistaken belief that they can obtain increased protection by massive doses of vitamin A.

Vitamin A and Convalescence

During infections the body uses up more vitamin A than in normal health. The stores of vitamin A in the body are depleted in the course of a long, chronic infection unless the supply in the diet is greater than normal. Although, as pointed out, massive doses taken during the infection will not achieve significant results in arresting the disease, a reasonable increase during convalescence will insure that recovery will not be retarded by a mild vitamin A deficiency. It is wise, therefore, during convalescence and for some time afterward, especially in growing children, to increase the vitamin intake above the amounts recommended for normal individuals. It may well be doubled. Where this cannot be done by diet alone, vitamin concentrates should be used.

These considerations regarding "anti-infectivity" and the requirement in the course of infections and convalescence hold not only for vitamin A, but also for the vitamin B complex and vitamins C and D. They are all required for growth and healthy development. To increase the vitamin supply by a reasonable amount—there is no need for massive doses— is a simple measure which may prevent an infection or a long convalescence from permanently retarding growth and development; it will certainly tend to curtail the harm.

Vitamin A and Liver Diseases

It has been already mentioned that the fat in the diet facilitates the passage from the intestine into the body of carotenoids, the vegetable form of vitamin A. Fat in the diet also tends to prevent the vitamin A from disappearing from the liver too quickly. When the amount of fat in the diet is restricted for long periods, there is a danger of vitamin A deficiency unless deliberate measures are taken to prevent it. This may account for the finding of an abnormally high incidence of vitamin A deficiency among people with cirrhosis of the liver, which is a chronic disease of the liver. The diets of patients with liver disease are commonly restricted with respect to fats. The possibility of vitamin A deficiency appears in these cases for three reasons: first, because the chief animal sources of this vitamin are eliminated by the restriction of fat; second, because the passage of carotenoids (the vegetable form of vitamin A) from the intestine into the body may be seriously interfered with by reason of the insufficiency of fat in the diet; and, third, because the vitamin A which is absorbed is either burned too quickly or not retained long enough because of the low-fat diet. If the liver is extensively damaged it secretes less bile into the intestine. This also will tend to diminish the amount of carotenoids which the intestine can absorb.

For these reasons people suffering from liver disease, whether acute or chronic, whether caused by bacteria or poisons, should obtain their vitamin A as vitamin A (from animal sources) and not as carotenoids from vegetables. Bile is not essential for the absorption of vitamin A. The richest sources of vitamin A are the fish-liver oils (halibut, cod). These are preferable to dairy products (milk and butter) as sources of vitamin A because in the latter, as already mentioned, part of the "vitamin A" is carotenoids.

Vitamin Deficiency and Kidney-Stone Formation

Experimental animals given a diet severely deficient in vitamin A and phosphorus frequently are found with stone in the kidney or ureter. Kidney stone is one of the oldest known human diseases. The finding in animals suggested that a mild but long-standing vitamin A deficiency might be one of the causes of stone in the kidney or ureter in human beings. Experimental and clinical studies have shown, however, that the trouble here is not that these people eat inadequate amounts of vitamin A. There is often an abundance of vitamin A in the diet, and administration of vitamin A concentrates does not improve the condition.

On the other hand an unduly high proportion of these patients were found with a subnormal recovery rate in the glare blindness test. In other words, the eyes of these people reacted as if they were not eating enough vitamin A. Yet when they were given large doses of vitamin A their rate of recovery in the glare blindness test remained subnormal.

It seems, therefore, that these patients suffer from some physiological disturbance which prevents their bodily chemistry from using vitamin A adequately. This disturbance contributes in some way to the formation of kidney (or ureter) stone. Unfortunately, there appears to be no hope of benefit or cure for them in taking vitamin A by mouth.

A Possible Explanation, a Hope, and a Moral

In some cases where the glare blindness test discloses an apparent vitamin A deficiency there is no recovery of normal vision after massive doses of vitamin A alone. But some of these special cases regained normal vision when, in addition to the vitamin A, large doses of the vitamin B complex were given.

Is it possible that sufferers from kidney stone may be relieved if they are given other vitamins as well as vitamin A?

There is a moral to be drawn here. Vitamins work best in co-operation.

CHAPTER V

The Vitamin B Complex, the Admirable Crichton of the Vitamins

Vitamin B: at Least Six Vitamins

IT IS unfortunate that vitamin B is not only the most difficult of the vitamins to describe and to understand, but also the most difficult to obtain in abundant quantities. It is not one vitamin but many. They occur together in natural products, yet the proportions of each vary from source to source. They are the most difficult to assay biologically with any precision. It has become necessary to speak of the different members of the B complex as distinctly different vitamins, because they are different chemical substances. Yet they are so complementary in their physiological action that we may eventually take up again the now discarded term "vitamin B" in describing the correlated action of this many-membered complex.

Vitamin B as a Tonic

Vitamin B is the modern, scientific substitute for the sulphur and molasses, bitters, and tonics of our grandmothers and the medical quacks of the last generation—with the difference that vitamin B, used intelligently, is effective. It is valuable in the treatment of such a variety of conditions as the neuritis of chronic alcoholism and of pregnancy, the nausea and sickness following massive irradiation with X-rays, constipation and intestinal pain, and even in some cases of chronic arthritis and heart disease. More important than any of these uses is the fact that it is a tonic even in well people. It stimulates without a letdown.

In the course of other studies, the author has received many unsolicited reports of this tonic effect. Housewives, for instance, found that doing their housework called for less effort than formerly; salesmen and teachers did not feel their usual fatigue at the end of the day. These people by customary standards were well people, but clearly they had not been getting enough "vitamin B" for abundant health. Their improvement resulted from a daily supplement of 1000 International Units of vitamin B_1 daily, taken in some form which also conveyed the rest of the vitamin B complex.

Climbing the Highest Mountain in the World without and with Vitamins

The tonic effect of vitamins B and C was demonstrated in the experience of the Mount Everest climbers. To reach the peak of Mount Everest, which is more than 29,000 feet high, has been the Great Adventure of British mountain climbers since about 1920. There have been seven attempts, all unsuccessful. It is a supreme test of skill, organization, and physical endurance.

Previous to the 1933 expedition all the climbers found that

at an altitude of 23,000 feet "almost any kind of food was unpalatable . . . and nauseating above that." This was thought to be an unavoidable effect of the high altitude.

For the 1933 expedition a nutrition expert was consulted, Dr. S. S. Zilva of the Lister Institute of London. He suggested a ration which was richer in vitamins as well as adequate in calories. One of the members of the expedition reported the result:

The painful spectacle was observed of climbers, who should have been languidly complaining of loss of appetite, in fact riotously demanding the commons of an ordinary robust Englishman at the altitude of London. This state of things prevailed even at 25,700 feet. It was only at 27,400 feet that a serious change occurred.

Even at this altitude F. S. Smythe, who went above 28,000 feet, wrote:

Our only grouse was the food. This had not worked according to plan. We craved for something more substantial than jellies and "slops." Shipton's constant plaint was, "Oh, for a few dozen eggs!" I sighed for a tin of Frankfurter sausages and sauerkraut. . . . Unfortunately the rations for high camps had naturally been based on previous experience.

The members of the 1933 expedition believed that their better appetites when they were high up on the mountain were due to the fact that they had deliberately acclimatized themselves to high altitudes more slowly than had the members of previous expeditions. But those who have experimented with vitamins will recognize in the experience of the pre-1933 expeditions a clear sign of deficiency in the vitamin B complex.

This is another example of man's inability to choose an

adequate diet instinctively. It is true that in the drawing up of a ration adequate for extreme conditions such as Mount Everest expeditions the experience of an old campaigner is of great value; but it must be supplemented by the knowledge of a student of scientific nutrition. It is nearly a century since Englishmen first made mountain climbing a serious sport. Yet in the mountaineering feat which calls for the greatest sustained effort the diet on the first expeditions was inadequate in quality. The difference in a diet good enough for the altitude of London or for one or two days' climbing in the Alps, and a diet which will sustain a man through the long trek on the high Tibetan plateau, followed by several weeks on Everest, is more than a matter of quantity—calories. The quality must be better; it must contain more vitamins, and probably also more animal protein. Hard and prolonged muscular work and a high-carbohydrate diet call for more than the normal intake of vitamins A, B, and C.

In this there is a lesson for everybody. A vitamin intake adequate for sustained great physical effort makes the performance of ordinary daily tasks easier. We are prepared, in this respect at least, against an unexpected emergency, of illness as well as of work. More important than this, we feel better, we are a little less tired at the end of the day, we have a little better time of it. For this purpose, with our diet as it is today, an increase in vitamin B is the most important addition we can make.

§1

Vitamin B₁ (Thiamine)

The best-known member of the B complex is, as its name implies, B_1. It is also known by its chemical name, thiamine chloride, or simply thiamine. More is known about it, its mode of action in the body, the signs of its deficiency, its chemistry and distribution in nature, than about any other member of the B complex.

Briefly, severe thiamine deficiency leads to a form of neuritis and general weakness called beri-beri or polyneuritis. (Its recognition and differentiation from other forms of neuritis are problems for the physician.) This disease occurs wherever polished rice is the main item of diet, or where white flour is eaten instead of whole cereal grains, and at the same time less milk is used. Beri-beri is a common occurrence in the Far East. In 1938, 60 per cent of all the cases admitted to St. Luke's Hospital in Shanghai had symptoms of beri-beri. The disease is also common in South America. It has been found in Louisiana. A few years ago there were twenty-five cases in a county jail in New Jersey. It is now appearing in Iceland, and cases of it occur regularly in Newfoundland and Labrador, where, during the winter and spring, the population lives very largely on a diet of white bread.

In the United States generally there is very little beri-beri. Its commonest occurrence is among chronic alcoholics. The trouble with the chronic alcoholic is that his diet is like the traditional Kentucky breakfast—a bottle of whisky, a juicy steak, and a bulldog (the bulldog to eat the steak). The chronic alcoholic lives, typically, on a diet of whisky, coffee, and sandwiches. He suffers from undernutrition and malnutrition. After a certain time on this regime he comes down with severe neuritis, in which there may be not only pain but also wrist-drop and failing spinal reflexes. He can be quickly relieved by thiamine, even when his consumption of alcohol is increased. But if he wishes to be really cured he needs nourishment of every category and psychological treatment.

Mild Vitamin B₁ Deficiency Is Widespread

Although there is little severe thiamine deficiency in America and Europe, a moderate deficiency of long duration is the most important nutritional problem for the populations of those areas. Nutrition surveys have shown that the average child and adult in the United States and England do not receive enough thiamine for the highest state of health. In children this deficiency causes subnormal growth and poor appetite.

In adults mild vitamin B deficiency is responsible for much of the constipation, flatulence, and dyspepsia characteristic of middle and old age. With this condition frequently go headaches, lack of stamina, and chronic fatigue. This whole complex of symptoms can in most cases be relieved (if there is no ulcer, tumor, or infection) by a good diet fortified by a daily supplement of 750/1000 International Units of thiamine and a liberal amount of the remainder of the B complex.

Thiamine Deficiency in Pregnancy, Severe Infections, and Heart Disease

When the thiamine intake is barely sufficient to prevent beri-beri, an additional stress on the body is likely to bring on the disease. Such, for instance, is the beri-beri of pregnancy. The former intake of thiamine is no longer sufficient after the strain of pregnancy is added. In southern India, where nearly all women suffer from vitamin B deficiency, premature births are three times as frequent as with the women of northern India, whose vitamin B intake is more nearly adequate. Neuritis of pregnancy (simply another name for beri-beri) occurs commonly enough in the United States.

An increase in the amount of physical work, infections with fever, hyperthyroidism—in fact, any condition in which there is an increase in metabolism[1] calls for more than the normal amount of thiamine. This important point is often overlooked in planning the diet of expeditions, of long camping trips, of soldiers, and even in hospitals.

Special attention should also be given to the vitamin B content of the diet in heart disease. Whenever neuritis is associated with enlargement of the heart, one may expect some degree of vitamin B deficiency. This is not always true, but the therapeutic test can be applied easily. That is, increase the vitamin B intake by large amounts[2]; if the diet is deficient in these vitamins, there will be a quick improvement of the heart condition and relief of the neuritis.

---

[1] Metabolism *means the total of the chemical and physical changes which go on in the body. It is estimated clinically by measuring the rate at which oxygen is used. The metabolic rate is usually defined in terms of calories, the amount of heat produced.*

[2] *From 10 to 50 milligrams daily. In order to administer such large amounts, the pure synthetic product must be used.*

Other Therapeutic Uses of Vitamin B

Many reports are coming into the current medical literature of relief of stubborn, obscure neuritic and arthritic pains through the use of rather large daily doses of vitamin B. The vitamin B complex is better here than one single component such as thiamine (vitamin B_1). If the patient has not received any lasting benefit from the treatment already prescribed, the vitamin B therapy deserves a trial. He should take 10 milligrams of thiamine daily, supplemented by liberal amounts of the vitamin B complex—4 to 6 teaspoonfuls daily of the best liquid concentrates. This treatment, which should continue three to six months, cannot possibly do any harm, and there is no objection to its use in conjunction with other forms of therapy.

Stimulation of Growth by Vitamins

So far, the importance of vitamins for growth has been mentioned only incidentally. All the vitamins are necessary for growth and healthy development. How much growth, how much health, depend, up to a certain limit, on the quantity of vitamins provided. Small amounts will prevent severe disease and insure some growth. To attain the maximum growth which the heritage of the child will permit, and to store up a capital of health which will last into a ripe and sound old age, a child must be provided with an abundance of vitamins. Few children today enjoy such an abundance.

This point was demonstrated experimentally by two California workers, Morgan and Barry. They worked with about one hundred children aged eleven and thirteen. The children were divided into two equal groups according to age and weight. All were somewhat undernourished; their weights at the beginning of the experiment ranged from 8 to 11 per cent subnormal.

The children in the first group were given each day two rolls weighing about three ounces, made of half white flour and half wheat germ. (Wheat germ is one of the good natural sources of the vitamin B complex.) The children in the second group were given two rolls of the same weight made of 100 per cent white flour. (Most of the vitamin B complex is removed in the milling of white flour.) Weight and height were measured periodically during the next three to four months. The children lived at home. No particular effort was made to influence their diet except that they were all given simple instruction in hygiene and nutrition.

The wheat-germ group averaged a gain of 0.35 pound per week, the white flour group only 0.14 pound. The wheat-germ group also made a greater gain in height, but the difference here was relatively smaller between the two groups.

The most interesting feature of this experiment is that the increase in growth can be attributed directly to the vitamin B complex (i.e., the wheat germ) which the children were fed. The two 50 per cent wheat-germ rolls provided about 200 International Units of vitamin B_1, plus other members of the B complex.

Vitamin B_1 Not Stored in the Body

One important question in connection with vitamins is the ability of the human body to lay up stores of them beyond its daily needs. Recently the author undertook to answer this question with regard to vitamin B_1. A number of healthy young men who had been living on a good diet were drafted into service as experimental animals. Daily they were given by intramuscular injection an additional 1000 to 10,000 units of vitamin B_1. In a few weeks they were so nearly saturated with the vitamin that they excreted in the urine 60 per cent of their daily intake. When they changed to a diet very low in vitamin B_1 and without daily injections, within a week the very small amounts of vitamin B_1 in the urine indicated that they were nearly depleted.

These findings on the storage and destruction of vitamin B_1 were completely confirmed by a later study. It occurred to the author that if the vitamin were made radioactive its position and progress in the human body could be traced accurately by physical methods. Radioactive B_1 was secured by substituting radioactive sulphur for ordinary sulphur in synthesizing the vitamin (sulphur is one of its components). The Geiger counter, a familiar piece of physical apparatus, is designed to give a click each time it receives an impulse emitted from the radioactive material being studied. The amount of radioactive material is measured by the number of clicks in a given time. So after the radioactive B_1 was administered to a young man who volunteered as an experimental subject, its vicissitudes in his body could be traced exactly by using a Geiger counter. By this method it was found that the vitamin is not only excreted rapidly, but is also rapidly destroyed in the body. About 10 per cent of the thiamine (vitamin B_1) in the body at any time is destroyed in the course of the next twenty-four hours. (The young man, incidentally, suffered no ill effects. In fact he stated that he felt all the better for the extra thiamine he had received. This was probably due to the exhilaration of the experiment.)

There is a similar excretion and destruction of vitamin C. These two vitamins are continually destroyed in the body and excreted in the urine, the amount in the urine being proportional to the amount taken in the preceding few days.

This inability of the human body to retain vitamins B_1 and C demands special attention to their provision on exploring expeditions, camping trips, and, in general, any situation where the normal food supply is restricted. Good concentrates of both vitamins are available for use in circumstances where difficulties of transport limit the food supply.

Human Requirements of Thiamine (Vitamin B_1)

Human requirements of thiamine cannot be stated as simply as some of the other vitamin requirements. The reason is that the amount of thiamine we need varies according to our weight and according to the amount we eat. This variation is illustrated in the table below, which gives, in relation to weight and diet, the minimum amount of thiamine necessary to prevent beri-beri (the thiamine-deficiency disease).

Weight	Total Calories in Daily Diet	Minimum Protective Intake of Thiamine (International Units Daily)
110 lbs.	2000	145
	3000	220
140 lbs.	2000	180
	3000	270
170 lbs.	2000	215
	3000	325
195 lbs.	2000	250
	3000	375
220 lbs.	2000	290
	3000	435
	3500	510

But as with the other vitamins, the minimum amount necessary to prevent deficiency disease is by no means enough for "buoyant" health. The author's studies of moderate vitamin B deficiency indicate that the thiamine requirement for a high level of health is four to five times the quantity needed to prevent beri-beri. That is, an adult should have 5 to 7 International Units of thiamine per pound of body weight per day. When metabolism is increased, whatever the cause—work, pregnancy, or disease—the requirement is greater in proportion to the increase in metabolism.

English students of this subject incline to the view that the thiamine content of the diet of their well-to-do classes is a good average figure for the normal requirement. This is about 450 International Units daily. Yet cases of beri-beri have been found among men who had been eating 400 units daily. In studying a large number of cases with gastrointestinal disturbances the author found that only about 25 per cent were relieved by an intake of 450–500 units, whereas about 75–80 per cent were markedly improved when the thiamine intake was increased by a daily supplement of 750–1000 units, accompanied by a corresponding amount of the remainder of the B complex.

All authorities agree that the requirement of growing children, relative to their body weight, is greater than that of adults. The daily requirement for children is about 10 International Units daily per pound of body weight.

Difficulty of Obtaining Enough Vitamin B

A good diet containing liberal amounts of salads, green vegetables, fresh fruit, milk, and meat provides daily about 500 International units of thiamine. The 750 to 1000 units daily recommended here are not obtained unless the matter is given some attention. The difficulty is that the foods commonly eaten do not contain high concentrations of thiamine. Another difficulty is the economic one. The tolerably palatable foods relatively rich in thiamine—fresh vegetables and fruit—are expensive. Vitamin B concentrates are prohibitively expensive for the poor. The provision of large amounts of vitamin B at a price which the low-income classes can afford, and in a form palatable enough for them to take day in and day out, calls for expert knowledge of nutrition, an educational campaign among growers, millers, and consumers, and possibly even some price control. It constitutes a major problem in nutritional engineering.

A Cheap Rich Source of Vitamin B

The problem of finding a cheap rich source of thiamine and the rest of the vitamin B complex can be solved by the use of a part of the wheat grain which millers call "the scalp of the sizings" or "middlings plus germ."

For the study of the effects of vitamin B on chronic dyspepsia it was necessary to obtain a cheap, palatable, and at the same time rich source of the whole B complex. Exploration among the flour mills revealed a fraction of the grain which is milled out in the process of making white flour. Most of this fraction was sold as animal feed; a little went into brown bread.

On analysis this fraction ("the scalp of the sizings") proved to contain most of the vitamin B in the grain; very little vitamin B is left in white flour. This cereal is probably the cheapest natural food source of the vitamin B complex. It contains three times the thiamine of the whole grain and has the same calorie and protein value. It can be cooked as porridge or baked into bread, muffins, scones, or other hot breads. For something under two cents per day per person it provides an optimum amount of vitamin B in palatable form.[3]

From inquiries made by the author it appears that to market this product, packaged and carrying some nationally advertised name, would probably increase the cost considerably. This is unnecessary. It can be obtained at any flour mill. The grocer can get it from the local miller if he makes the proper inquiries and is a little persistent.[4]

---

[3] *Since the distribution of this cereal to our patients began, its sale has grown in a remarkable way. Without a word of public advertising, simply by word-of-mouth recommendation, as much as 3000 to 5000 pounds is now sold for human consumption each week in Pasadena and Los Angeles.*

[4] *Some physicians have expressed to the author the fear that this product may contain too much roughage for some of their patients. In the author's experience with several hundred cases suffering from "colitis" and "irritable bowel" there were very few who could not tolerate as much as a quarter-pound of this cereal daily.*

Bread and Flour: The Best Part Thrown Away

Bread, "the Staff of Life"! This was true once upon a time. Bread made of whole-wheat flour was formerly for the poor, who lived mainly on bread, their most important source of vitamin B. But bread is only a filler now, a source of calories (at about twice the cost of sugar) and of some second-rate protein.

The public has been led to prefer highly milled white flour and bread made from it. The following table shows the vitamin B_1 (thiamine) that has been lost.

Percentage of the Whole Grain in the Flour	Percentage of the Vitamin B_1 of the Whole Grain Which Remains	Vitamin B_1 in a Slice of Bread Made from This Flour (International Units)
100 whole-wheat flour	100	30
75	27	8.2
70 (flour used in making white bread)	20	7.5
60	15	4.5
55	12	3
50	7	2.1
40 cake and pastry flour	0	0

In the light of such figures as these, some authorities have strongly recommended our eating only whole-wheat bread. But this procedure would have several disadvantages.

In the United States, at any rate, it is a significant disadvantage that whole-wheat bread does not toast as well as white. Countless Americans would rebel at the prospect of starting their day with anything but the customary white-bread toast. Another disadvantage is that whole-grain meal does not keep as well as white flour; nor does whole-wheat bread keep as well as white. For these reasons, whole-wheat bread is ill suited to large-scale modern baking and distribution.

In any case, the substitution of whole-wheat bread for white bread would not make a significant difference in America. Our survey indicated that in southern California the daily consumption of bread and rolls is only about one-quarter pound per person. At the level at which bread is eaten in England, whole-wheat bread alone would supply nearly enough vitamin B_1 to prevent beri-beri. In the United States, however, with a much lower per capita bread consumption, only 100 International Units would be obtained this way.

In July 1940, the English government decided to fortify white flour with crystalline thiamine in such quantities that the daily per capita intake of that vitamin will be increased by approximately 100 International Units. This is a very significant decision for a number of reasons. For the first time in the history of the world the government of a great country has recognized by law the necessity of supplying a vitamin as well as simply gross food for the whole population. Equally important is the recognition by a government that dietary improvement by the educational process is slow and haphazard. Thirdly, a government has embraced the principle of fortification of a staple foodstuff for a whole nation. In other words, the nutrition of a whole nation is to be improved by plan and measure without calling on the individuals of that nation to do anything.

Other Sources of Vitamin B_1

Various other solutions have been suggested for the problem of obtaining enough vitamin B_1 for the population at an accessible price. One is to mix white flour with finely ground rice bran, which contains about 250 International units of thiamine per ounce. Pure wheat germ, which is yellow and flaky, has also been recommended. It is rich in thiamine, but it is unpalatable, it keeps poorly, and it is expensive if enough of it is taken to meet the optimum requirement of 750–1000 International Units per day.

The richest source of the whole vitamin B complex is brewer's yeast. Dried, it contains 500–700 International Units of thiamine per ounce. But it is relatively expensive, and in the opinion of most people highly unpalatable.

The Value of Peanut Butter

Peanut butter is the Cinderella among foods. It is good, and its calorie value is high. It is rich in carbohydrates and fats (unlike Cinderella); it contains somewhat more protein than beef. And it is among the very best food sources of vitamin B; an ounce (two tablespoonfuls) contains about 125 International Units of thiamine. It is cheap, and most children are fond of it.

Peanut butter is a boon to mothers who must make up lunches every day. A pint of milk (preferably "vitamin D" milk), whole-wheat bread peanut-butter sandwiches, and a tomato or an orange make a nearly perfect lunch from the

nutritional point of view. It is doubtful if another lunch
could be devised which would be as cheap and nearly as good.

How Necessary Are Vegetables?

One can nearly always raise an argument about the
necessity of vegetables. Women are usually "For"; men and
children, "Against." The table of vitamin contents of foods
at the end of the book shows that even liberal amounts of
vegetables will not supply the amount of thiamine recommended here.

Then why bother at all, especially with spinach? To be
honest, spinach cannot be defended today with the ardor
of a few years ago. The *New Yorker* a while back printed
what has become the spinach classic. A little boy is pictured
indignantly rejecting a plate offered to him with the words:
"It's broccoli, dear." His famous reply is: "I say it's spinach,
and I say the hell with it!"

As far as spinach is concerned, he was on strong ground.
We know now that none of the calcium it contains and only
about half of its iron can be used by the body.

It may be true that a diet containing even liberal amounts
of fresh vegetables, fresh meat, and milk will probably not
furnish enough vitamin B for the highest state of health.
Nevertheless, the amount obtained in this way is enough to
keep one well protected against beri-beri. The additional
50 per cent necessary for "buoyant" health can then be
obtained easily from the "scalp of the sizings" for breakfast,
brewer's yeast (beer, alas, will not do), or a small amount of
some vitamin B concentrate.

There are even better arguments in favor of vegetables.

Except spinach, they supply indispensable minerals. They also insure that the proteins will be a mixture, which is essential. And they provide vitamin A, the rest of the B complex, vitamin C, and undoubtedly others which have not yet been discovered. Finally, most people will not take the trouble to secure the special cereal product we have described above, nor brewer's yeast, nor vitamin B concentrates. For them, vegetables, with fresh meat and milk, are the chief sources of vitamins and minerals.

Fruit, Meat, and Milk as Sources of Vitamin B_1

The banana deserves a place of honor as a source of vitamins in infant feeding where the food budget is limited. One banana contains 28 International Units of thiamine and a fair amount of vitamin C. On the other hand, it is not specially useful in adult diets; as the main source of vitamins it would supply too much carbohydrate for grown people. The other common fruits—apples, peaches, pears, and the melons —cost too much in proportion to their richness as sources of either thiamine or other members of the B complex. One cannot eat enough of them to improve one's vitamin B intake materially.

Fresh meat is a time-honored, somewhat overrated standby. One quarter-pound of fresh lean beef contains about 50 International Units of thiamine. Fowl and pork are much richer in this respect than beef. Liver is not much superior to ordinary cuts as far as thiamine is concerned, but it is richer in other components of the B complex, in iron, and in an important anti-anemic principle. Apart from such considerations as flavor and tenderness, beef liver is as good as calf liver.

Milk is an important source of vitamin B; for infants it is the most important source. Raw whole milk contains about 75 International Units of thiamine per pint. There is little lost in pasteurization. Most evaporated and dried milks contain nearly all the original vitamin B content.

Thiamine (Vitamin B₁) in Whisky, Why Not in Milk?

Recently there has been talk of adding thiamine to whisky. As a means of protecting chronic alcoholics from alcoholic neuritis this would no doubt be a laudable undertaking. But for widespread general benefit the addition of thiamine to milk deserves a great deal more consideration and support.

Milk could be made a first-class food simply by the addition of a minute amount of thiamine and other members of the vitamin B complex now available commercially in crystalline form at low price. Fresh cow's milk naturally contains about 150 International Units of thiamine per quart. One-tenth of an ounce of crystalline thiamine added to 250 gallons of milk would provide an enrichment of 800 International Units per quart. Crystalline thiamine is now so cheap when bought in large quantities that this supplement need add only one-third of a cent per quart to the cost.

Vitamin B Concentrates

Several good vitamin B concentrates are now on the market. Although they are too expensive to be used by most families as the staple source, they are valuable when it is desirable to administer large doses in a short time. They are useful on long camping trips, expeditions into wild or barren country, and whenever vegetables, fruit, and milk are taken along in the dry form in order to reduce the bulk to be carried. In buying vitamin B concentrates the purchaser should compute how many units he is getting at the price and buy that product which gives him the most units for the money.

Crystalline Thiamine (Vitamin B_1)

Synthetic crystalline thiamine is now on the market in tablet form and in solution ready for injection. It is useful where there is a severe vitamin B_1 deficiency, as in alcoholic neuritis and the neuritis of pregnancy. It can be given in massive doses by intravenous or intramuscular injection to bring the patient quickly out of a critical state. A patient who has been proved to be deficient in thiamine is almost certainly deficient in other members of the vitamin B complex. Thiamine cannot replace these, and they also must be provided.

Loss of Vitamin B in Cooking

Though you may be careful to get vitamins in the market, you can still lose them very easily in the kitchen. Too often in the cooking of vegetables most of the vitamin B and other water-soluble vitamins are thrown out in the cooking water. The same applies to canned vegetables. Canned and strained spinach, for instance, contains only about one-fourth the vitamin B originally in the fresh leaves.

It is advisable to cook vegetables with a minimum of water, and not to throw away the water. Using it may tax the cook's ingenuity, but it is worth the trouble. The water contains not only the water-soluble vitamins but also important minerals. Two other principles are to be borne in mind in the cooking of vegetables. One is that soda should never be used; it may give vegetables a prettier color, but it destroys the vitamins in part. The other is that, as far as possible, air should be excluded during cooking. For this reason a pressure-cooker or double boiler is preferable to an open pot.

Restaurant Food

The last point is especially important for those who obtain most of their meals in restaurants or wherever the food is kept warm for hours, spread out on steam-tables. Under these conditions a large proportion of the vitamin content of meat and vegetables is lost. Those who must obtain their meals in such places are exposed to the danger of vitamin deficiencies, even though they may believe themselves protected because they eat vegetables. Uncooked vegetables and to a lesser extent fruit salads are some safeguards. (See table, pages 170 and 171.)

§2

Vitamin B₁ and Horticulture

During the past year or two the use of vitamin B_1 in horticulture has been widely publicized. It has produced some very gratifying results under controlled conditions in plant-physiology laboratories. It has also been found to be sometimes beneficial in a few kinds of ordinary gardening; for instance, in rooting cuttings of certain plants and in preventing retarded growth when trees and shrubs are transplanted. But successful results vary greatly according to the type of plant and the character of the soil. At the present time extensive studies are being made to determine precisely the horticultural conditions under which the gardener can count on getting the desired results from vitamin B_1. Until these studies are completed the use of vitamin B_1 in gardening must be largely haphazard. Try it, if you like, but do not be disappointed if nothing happens. Certainly vitamin B_1 is not a horticultural cure-all.

Vitamin B₂ (G, Flavin, Riboflavin)

If we reversed the United States motto "*E Pluribus Unum*," we would have a good description of the vitamin B complex.

In 1926 it was proved that what had been called vitamin B was more than one substance. A division was then made between vitamin B_1, the antineuritic factor now called thiamine, and the remainder, which was called B_2. About ten years later, B_2 was shown to consist of at least four factors. For one of these, whose chemical nature was established at that time, the designation B_2 was appropriated. It is also called vitamin G, flavin, and riboflavin.

Vitamin B_2 of course is essential for growth. As it is a part of one of the mechanisms whereby food materials are burned in the body, we can reasonably guess that it exercises an important function in the adult as well as in the growing child.

Vitamin B_2 Deficiency Diseases

In the past two years it has been discovered that a definite disease can be produced experimentally by a vitamin B_2 deficient diet and then cured by adding this vitamin in the pure state to such a diet. This disease is called *cheilosis;* a name suggested as being more accurate is *ariboflavinosis* (which means "without riboflavin").

The characteristic signs are reddening and cracking of the skin at the angles of the mouth. The lips and tongue are abnormally red; there is a greasy shedding of the skin at the folds between the nostrils and cheeks; and the corners of the eyes and the underside of the eyelids may be involved.

For many years this disease was overlooked or confused with other diseases such as pellagra. It is now recognized as quite common in the southern United States, where in certain regions it may be even more prevalent than pellagra.

It is not rare farther north. In one New York clinic a case turns up about once a month.

There is a growing accumulation of evidence that vitamin B_2 is necessary for the health of the eyes. Thus, cataracts have been observed in rats, mice, chickens, and monkeys that were maintained on a vitamin B_2 deficient diet. The cataract involves the lens of the eye. Addition of the vitamin to the diet will not repair the damage that has already occurred, but it will arrest the further progress of the disease.

There is so far no proof that the formation of cataracts in human beings is a vitamin-deficiency disease. The animal experiments are suggestive; cataract formation in human beings is a degenerative change; and it is known that the onset of senile degenerative changes in other human tissues is postponed or arrested by vitamin-rich diets. In India, where millions live on rations in which the vitamin intake and the quantity of food are low, cataracts are extremely frequent early in life. When some of these people were given additions of vitamin B_2 (and other vitamins) the further development of the cataracts was arrested.

In experimental animals in which vitamin B_2 deficiency has produced cataract, a diseased condition of the outer lining of the eyeball has been observed. A similar condition— but without the cataract—occurs in undernourished women toward the end of pregnancy. There are visual disturbances, burning sensations and excessive watering of the eyes, and failing vision. Unlike cataract, this condition can be cured by adding abundant amounts of vitamin B_2 to the diet.

In Chapter IV we mentioned that some individuals suffering from glare blindness and defective vision in dim light are not cured, as are the majority of these cases, by treatment with vitamin A. Many of these exceptional cases respond promptly, however, when vitamin B_2 is administered as well. At the same time, the inflammation of the eyeball (conjunctivitis) commonly present also subsides.

Human Requirements of Vitamin B_2

The human vitamin B_2 requirement has not yet been accurately determined. Provisionally it has been set at 1.5 milligrams daily for children under five years; 2 to 3 milligrams daily for adults.

Where vitamin B_2 deficiency disease is suspected, several times the above quantities should be administered. The vitamin can be purchased in the pure state at reasonable prices and in a form suitable for intravenous injection, if that is necessary. There is no danger of overdosage. Diagnosis and treatment of this or any other deficiency, however, should not be attempted by the layman.

Vitamin B_2 in Foods

The distribution of vitamin B_2 is on the whole similar to that of vitamin B_1, except that cereals—wheat and rice, for example—are not good sources. The best source is again yeast (baker's or brewer's), with 0.25 milligram per ounce. Taking into account the quantities which can be eaten in an ordinary diet, the next-best source is cow's milk, which contains 0.60 milligram per pint. Milk is the chief source of this vitamin in the dietary of children. There is no significant loss in pasteurization. Human milk contains only one-third the amount of B_2 in cow's milk and is therefore an inadequate source. It is remarkable that human milk is low in the vitamin one of whose outstanding effects is the promotion of growth.

One egg contains 0.25 milligram.

Almost as important as cow's milk and eggs as sources of B_2 are the green leafy vegetables. Beet greens, turnip greens, carrot tops, broccoli (flowers and leaves), are the richest. Spinach, lettuce, and cabbage are half as rich or less.

Soy beans (dried) are a very rich source. Other varieties of beans contain only one-tenth as much.

The best animal sources are liver and kidney. Next in order of potency are heart and ordinary cuts of beef, pork, and veal.

Vitamin B_2 is less affected by heat than B_1. On the other hand, it is destroyed by both visible and ultraviolet light. The same precautions in cooking and the use of the cooking water should be taken with this vitamin as with vitamin B_1.

§3

Nicotinic Acid and Pellagra

Pellagra is a nutritional deficiency disease of the poor in those regions in the United States, Italy, Egypt, and elsewhere where corn forms a large part of the diet. It has been estimated that there are more than 400,000 cases in the United States, mainly in the South.

The typical hillbilly is a good picture of chronic pellagra. In one of our large national magazines the hillbilly joke is frequently the best in the issue. But we could dispense with this source of humor if at the same time we could get rid of the most serious deficiency disease in the United States. If pellagra is left to develop unchecked, the mortality is nearly 70 per cent. In severe cases the mind is affected. Ten per cent of the inmates of mental institutions in the South are pellagrins.

For some time it has been known that pellagra is a deficiency disease and that a properly balanced diet would prevent it. But it has been extraordinarily difficult to put this knowledge into practice and change the diet of the poor in the pellagra regions. The inertia of ignorance is one great hindrance. Another, perhaps even more serious, is that the people are too poor to buy what they ought to eat.[5]

In the autumn of 1937 it was found that either one of two well-known chemicals, nicotinic acid and nicotinic acid amide, given in half-gram daily doses would quickly relieve severe cases of pellagra. It was already known that nicotinic acid is present in yeast and other rich sources of the vitamin B complex which had been successfully used to cure and prevent pellagra.

A very simple solution of the pellagra problem seemed to be available at last. Apparently all that was necessary was to distribute nicotinic acid in pills or capsules, or add it to salt. Besides ease of distribution, there was a further advantage in that nicotinic acid is a relatively cheap chemical, which no doubt will become cheaper with increasing demand.

In the summer of 1938, however, these hopes appeared to

---

[5] *Recently the Federal Writers' Project published a large number of brief autobiographies of Southerners, mostly tenant farmers and mill hands* (These Are Our Lives, University of North Carolina Press). *These accounts contain a good deal of incidental information about diet in that part of the Southern population which is just on the economic margin or below. For instance, when one man recalls his father "comin' in at the end of the day all tired out and eatin' our scant meal of cornbread, peas, and cane sirup," he is describing just the sort of diet that produces pellagra.*

When one reads in many of these accounts the weekly wages that must support a family, it is easy to understand why the diet is so bad.

be dashed. It was reported then that nicotinic acid alone gives only temporary relief from the symptoms of pellagra. After four to six weeks the symptoms return with their former severity. On the other hand, a permanent cure can be effected by eating daily about ⅕ of a pound of dried brewer's yeast or from one to two ounces of brewer's yeast with 1/1000 of an ounce of nicotinic acid.

The explanation of these apparently conflicting results is now clear. Pellagra as it is found in the field is most frequently a multiple-deficiency disease. The diet of pellagrins is seriously deficient in vitamins B_1, B_2, and nicotinic acid; insufficient amounts of first-class protein may be a contributory factor.

To treat pellagra successfully, therefore, the whole vitamin B complex must be provided in adequate amounts, plus some first-class protein. In terms of ordinary foodstuffs this means a diet of meat, milk, eggs, fresh green vegetables, and fruit. But this is a relatively expensive diet, far beyond the purse, the education, and the eating habits of the poor white and the poor Negro of the tenant farms and mill towns of the South.

An easy, economical solution is available and crying out for application. Since most of the vitamin B complex is being manufactured synthetically, these vital substances could easily be added to flour, cornmeal, and sugar as part of the processing. If this were done on a national scale, the cost would be small compared to the benefits that would result. Certainly the expense would be less than the present charge of maintaining pellagra clinics and dispensaries, providing hospitalization for pellagrins, and caring for thousands of cases of pellagrous insanity in public asylums.

The fortification of staple foods would prevent pellagra in its early mild stages and cure it without the individual's knowing it. To paraphrase the old Austrian joke, "Victory unavoidable, send the Crown Prince," the prevention and cure of pellagra would be unavoidable, indeed automatic, provided only that the individual ate enough to keep himself alive.

The beneficial consequences—economic, social, and political—for the whole United States cannot be overestimated.

Nicotinic Acid and Delirium Tremens

We have already mentioned alcoholic beri-beri, which is the result of a severe thiamine deficiency. Sometimes in addition to suffering the neuritis characteristic of this disease, the patient collapses in delirium tremens. The administration of thiamine does not help this second condition, and its consequences are frequently fatal. Recently, however, it has been found that the administration of large amounts of nicotinic acid—as in the treatment of pellagra—brings complete relief from the delirium in 24 to 48 hours. These people are actually suffering from a multiple-deficiency disease; they have both beri-beri and pellagra in a very acute state. The delirium tremens may be considered a form of acute pellagrous insanity.

Nicotinic Acid and Trench Mouth

There are recent reports from England that trench mouth, which is in itself a bacterial disease, can be cured by large doses of nicotinic acid. The explanation is interesting and instructive as showing how a vitamin deficiency, even though it may not be so severe as to cause the characteristic deficiency disease, may create a condition which favors another disease. In a healthy mouth the organisms which cause trench mouth are harmless. A mild nicotinic acid deficiency, however, lowers the resistance of the tongue tissue so that the organisms can invade it successfully and cause the disease.

§4

Vitamin B_6 (Pyridoxin)

Vitamin B_6 was isolated in crystalline form early in 1938. It is now manufactured and is on the market.

Vitamin B_6 deficiency is still for the most part a laboratory phenomenon. The deficiency is responsible for a characteristic disease of the skin and hair in rats, a form of anemia in dogs, and possibly diseases of the central nervous system.

So far, no characteristic vitamin B_6 deficiency disease in man has been proved. Because B_6 deficiency causes a skin disease in rats, this vitamin is being tried in a variety of chronic human skin diseases, but, pending further evidence, no precise statements can be made about how it can best be used.

In conjunction with other vitamins (B_1 and E), B_6 appears to be useful in the treatment of certain degenerative diseases of the human nervous system.

A number of physicians and the author have observed a marked "tonic" effect following the administration of this vitamin in very large doses—50 to 100 milligrams daily.

It is too early yet to appraise these results. There can be little doubt, however, that vitamin B_6 is necessary for human nutrition.

The occurrence of this vitamin in natural foodstuffs is in general the same as that of the other members of the B complex. This is not fortuitous. Soon after the vitamins of the B complex became available in the pure state, it was found that they are necessary for the growth of all forms of life—bacteria, protozoa, fungi, and higher plants, as well as the higher animals.

Crude cane molasses is a good source of vitamin B_6; beet molasses, on the other hand, is practically devoid of it. The branny coats of the cereal grains are also good sources; and it is present, of course, in relatively high concentration in yeast. In general, as sources of B_6, fruits and vegetables are poor; fish and meat are fair; seeds, legumes, and cereals are relatively rich.

§5

Pantothenic Acid

Pantothenic acid is the most recent member of the vitamin B complex to be isolated, its structure determined, and its manufacture undertaken. Its discovery came from two converging but originally independent lines of investigation. One line of investigation demonstrated that pantothenic acid is necessary for the growth of yeast and some bacteria; the other showed that it is essential for the growth of chicks and that its deficiency produces in them a characteristic disease of the skin and plumage.

The discovery of this vitamin is too recent for anything to be known of its specific role in human nutrition. As with the other members of the B complex, it almost certainly is necessary.

§6

Other Members of the Vitamin B Complex

We know that there are two more members of the vitamin B complex waiting to be chemically identified. Probably there will be still others. Recent reports suggest that for the man in the street who is not suffering from beri-beri or pellagra these unidentified vitamins (or they in conjunction with known vitamins) may prove to be even more important than the members of the B complex already identified.

For example, black-haired rats turn gray when kept on certain deficient diets. The precise nature of the deficiency is not clear yet; but it almost certainly involves one or more members of the B complex.

The reader must be warned that there is little likelihood of finding here any cure for silver threads among the gold (or brown). On the other hand, it would be too conservative to state that this has nothing whatever to do with the graying of human hair. There are a number of observations—the author's among them—which indicate that something may come of this. One thing, however, is certain—no vitamin yet known or suspected will cure baldness.

The study of the "anti-gray-hair factor," as it is called, while interesting enough for its own sake, has acquired an augmented importance with the discovery that a degeneration of the adrenal glands in rats is sometimes produced by the same diet that causes graying of their hair. The adrenal gland is essential to life, and its degeneration is involved in the process of senility. Do we have here, then, a clue to the existence of a vitamin which, administered in massive doses, could retard the onset of senility? We can only hope, as we wait for the results of further investigations of the anonymous members of the vitamin B complex.

CHAPTER VI

Vitamin C,
the Preventive of Scurvy

Scurvy—a Vitamin C Deficiency Disease

SCURVY is an ancient disease. Although empirical cures for it appeared as early as the 1600's, its real cause—vitamin C deficiency—was not discovered until the twentieth century. Today the knowledge of how to prevent and cure it by vitamin C is a commonplace in the medical schools. This chapter in medical history is apparently finished—until the next discovery, which may have been announced even before these lines are printed.

The story of scurvy should be so well known that the disease will disappear from civilized communities even in its mildest forms. All that is required is that we know the common antiscorbutic foods, and that the manufacturers of synthetic vitamin C sell it at a much lower price than they do now (which they can well afford). Synthetic vitamin C should be sold in grocery stores as well as drug stores.

Scurvy was common in Europe in modern times until the introduction of the potato into the ordinary diet. Although this vegetable was introduced into England in 1585, it was still a luxury in 1650; and it did not begin to be cultivated on a large scale until the latter part of the eighteenth century. The disease then disappeared even among the poor. It has reappeared on a large scale only when there has been a failure of the potato crop, as in Ireland in 1847 and in Norway in 1914.

One of the most interesting chapters in the history of scurvy could be constructed from the records of the British Navy and merchant marine in the eighteenth century. Scurvy was practically an occupational disease among seamen on long voyages. A few naval surgeons and ship captains, though they were mistaken about the causes of the disease, managed to hit on effective remedies and preventives.

Captain James Cook, the circumnavigator, was particularly conscientious about the health of his crew. His success in preventing scurvy is recorded in the entry in his *Journal* for Thursday, April 13, 1769. On that day his ship had reached Tahiti after a voyage of about seven months.

The Ship's company had in general been very healthy, owing in a great measure to the Sour kroutt, Portable Soup and Malt; the two first were served to the People [i.e., the crew], the one on Beef Days and the other on Banyan Days. Wort was made of the Malt, and at the discretion of the Surgeon given to every man that had the least simptoms of Scurvy upon him. By this means, and the Care and Vigilance of Mr. Monkhouse, the Surgeon, this disease was prevented from getting a footing in the Ship. The Sour Kroutt, the Men at first would not eat it, until I put it in practice—a method I never once Knew to fail with seamen—and this was to have some of it dressed every day for the Cabin Table, and permitted all the Officers, without exception, to make use of it, and left it to the Option of the men either to take as much as they pleased or none at all; but this practice was not continued above a week before I found it necessary to put every one on board to an allowance; for such are the tempers and disposition of Seamen in general that whatever you give them out of the common way—altho' it be ever so much for their good— it will not go down, and you will hear nothing but murmurings against the Man that first invented it; but the moment they see their superiors set a value upon it, it becomes the finest stuff in the world and the inventor an honest fellow.[1]

The practice of calling an English sailor a "limey" is a linguistic relic of another attempt to prevent scurvy among seamen. As early as 1600 the crew of a British ship, during a four-month voyage from England to Bombay, were kept from scurvy by a ration of lemon juice. Similar uses of it are recorded sporadically through the eighteenth century. Finally, in 1804, the British Navy made a regular issue of lemon juice compulsory. The juice of the Mediterranean lemon was used, but it was generally called "lime" juice. Hence the ships in which it was rationed out were called "lime-juicers" and the sailors "limeys."

For the next fifty years after 1804, scurvy was a comparatively rare disease in the British Navy. The rest of the story is not so happy. About the middle of the nineteenth century, West Indian lime juice was gradually substituted for lemon juice. Political factors were partly responsible. The antiscorbutic value of the lemon was thought to be in its acidity, and the West Indian lime was fully as acid as the lemon. Unfortunately, however, it contains much less vitamin C. When scurvy reappeared after the substitution of lime juice, the result, unhappily, was the drawing of the wrong conclusion and the discrediting of citrus juice generally as a preventive of scurvy.

---

[1] *Captain W. J. L. Wharton, R.N., F.R.S., ed.,* Captain Cook's Journal during His First Voyage round the World in H.M. Bark "Endeavour," 1768–71, London, *1893*.

This illustrates the kind of difficulty which for a long time prevented eradication of the disease. All sorts of wrong clues were followed up, all sorts of mistaken inferences drawn. Scurvy at sea was blamed on sea air, cold, and the eating of salt meat. In more recent times, the poisons from putrefying meat and fish (1900) and bacteria (1904, 1916) were held responsible. Scurvy has been attributed to a decrease of alkalinity in the blood. In 1917 constipation was put forward as the cause. Infantile scurvy, which appeared about the middle of the nineteenth century as patent baby-foods replaced mother's milk among the middle and upper classes, was not even correctly diagnosed until toward the end of the century.

This is not to say that there were no investigators on the right track. But erroneous and correct views held the field on an equal basis until Holst and his colleagues in 1907–1912 proved definitely that scurvy is the result of deficiency in a specific substance—vitamin C. The identification of this effective agent in antiscorbutic foods was actively pursued from 1907 on, culminating in the artificial synthesis of vitamin C in 1933.

The problems remaining now are chiefly two: one is clinical—recognition of the disease in its earliest stages; the other is less a problem than an educational task—the prevention of the disease. People must be taught that prolonged hard muscular work, severe climatic cold, and infections call for more than normal amounts of vitamin C. In outfitting expeditions and provisioning long voyages, in drawing up the food ration of lumber camps and troops in the field, the increased requirement of vitamin C (and of vitamins A and B as well) must be taken into account.

Special measures must also be taken with patients who

are kept on very restricted diets. For example, people suffering from gastric or duodenal ulcer, diabetes, or allergic diseases are often advised by their physicians to give up fresh vegetables and fruit juices. This obviously paves the way for scurvy and other vitamin-deficiency diseases. Even now reports appear in the medical literature of cases being treated for duodenal ulcer which develop scurvy and beriberi (vitamin B_1 deficiency). In such cases the vitamin intake must be kept up to the required amount by doses of vitamin concentrates or synthetic vitamins.

Signs of Scurvy

The signs of early or "latent" scurvy in children are a subnormal rate of growth, a tendency to bleed easily, some anemia, and a lowered resistance to infection. These symptoms in themselves are not diagnostic of scurvy. They may be the result of a concomitant vitamin B deficiency; vitamins B and C are water-soluble and their distribution among fruits and vegetables, apart from the citrus fruits, runs parallel. The diagnosis of latent scurvy can be made only by a physician trained in the laboratory methods of vitamin chemistry.

There is no scurvy in babies before four and one-half months. Later, they are prone to severe scurvy. When it occurs, the onset is between the sixth and ninth months. There is pallor, wasting, and the child is reluctant to move because of pain; the limbs are swollen and discolored; the child is fretful, with a rapid pulse and breathing. Hemorrhage of the gums may appear if the teeth have come through; this is one of the late signs of the disease. These children cry when anyone comes near for fear of being touched or moved, movement is so painful.

In adults the signs of latent scurvy are, as in children, a tendency to bleed easily, anemia, and lowered resistance to infection. Later there is loss in weight, progressive weakness, and pallor. In manifest (severe) scurvy the gums become swollen and bleed easily, the teeth become loose and fall out; a slight bruise causes extensive bleeding under the skin. The skin is dry and rough, and numerous spots of bleeding appear under the skin on the legs, arms, and trunk.

This dreadful condition is quickly cured by 1/1500 of an ounce of vitamin C daily! Manifest scurvy is rare now. By prescribing citrus and tomato juices for babies at an early age, the pediatricians have practically eradicated it in children. On the average American diet it rarely, if ever, occurs in adults. But it does appear occasionally among people who for various reasons have been living for long periods on an inadequate diet. There was an outbreak of scurvy, for instance, in Maine as recently as 1938. It appears in Newfoundland and Labrador as a consequence of the poor-quality winter diet. It flared up a number of times among prisoners of war in the years 1914–1918. And in Vienna, in the dreadful period immediately following the end of the war, it was widespread among the children of the poor.

Human Requirements of Vitamin C

Pure crystalline vitamin C is now sold in nearly all drug stores. It is usually the artificially synthesized product. For this and other reasons it is more useful to describe the daily human requirement in terms of milligrams rather than in International units. (One milligram of the pure substance is equivalent to 20 International units of vitamin C.)

Ten milligrams of vitamin C daily will protect a young baby from scurvy. The breast-fed baby probably receives four to five times this amount in the mother's milk. The rapidly growing child requires more than this amount of vitamin C for a good rate of growth and health. Three to four milligrams daily per pound of body weight until 100–150 milligrams are being taken is a liberal but not an excessive amount. A tumblerful of orange juice supplies rather more than this.

For adults, 40 milligrams daily—about three ounces of orange juice—are more than enough to prevent scurvy. The optimal amount, however, is approximately one milligram per pound of body weight per day.

Vitamin C in Fruit Juices

By far the best common sources of vitamin C are the citrus fruit juices—orange, lemon, and grapefruit. These three citrus fruits are, weight for weight, equally potent. The edible portion of one medium-sized orange contains about 60 milligrams of ascorbic acid (vitamin C). Orange juice is equally potent whether fresh, properly canned, or chilled and frozen. But oranges in storage lose some of their potency. No precise figure can be given, but from the available data it appears that about 40 per cent of the potency is lost in a month's storage. Hence, if the reader gets his oranges from a stored supply—and this is almost certainly so at any distance from the orange-growing regions—he should increase his ration of orange juice enough to compensate for this 40 per cent loss in storage.

Orange and lemon peel on the basis of weight are twice to three times as potent as the juice. But marmalade is negligible as a source of vitamin C. Even if most of the vitamin were not lost in cooking, only an individual with a superhuman marmalade capacity could eat enough to do him any good.

Tomato juice has about half the vitamin C content of the citrus juices; the canned juice is as good as the fresh.

Dr. Sidebotham and Pine-needle Tea

During the Alaska gold rush an American physician, Dr. Sidebotham, found himself with a number of scurvy cases on his hands and none of the standard antiscorbutics—fresh fruit and vegetables—anywhere within several hundred miles. The only green thing available was pine-needles. So, on speculation, he made a decoction by extracting pine-needles with an equal quantity of water. Under this treatment his patients recovered. Later investigations showed that this decoction contains almost as much vitamin C as orange juice. There is little likelihood that this pine-needle brew will ever replace orange juice in general diet, but the knowledge may be useful some time in an emergency. There are reports that it is used in the U.S.S.R.

Vitamin C in Other than Citrus Fruits

Most fresh fruits contain some vitamin C. The amount differs in the same fruit according to variety. Storage cuts it down. If an apple a day keeps the doctor away, it does not do so by virtue of the amount of vitamin C it contains. And 40 per cent of the originally low vitamin content of apples is lost when they are stored for eight months at a temperature a little above freezing (that is, kept in cold storage). With nearly all non-citrus fruits, the quantity that can be included in the ordinary diet furnishes too little vitamin C to be worth considering.

An exception must be made, however, for a few fruits. Strawberries, raspberries, and gooseberries are excellent sources; on the basis of fresh weight they are about half as rich as orange juice. Except at the height of their season, though, they are uneconomical in comparison with other equally good sources of vitamin C.

Melons also are good sources, especially in view of the quantity in an ordinary serving. The juice is about one-fifth as rich in vitamin C as orange juice. Dried watermelon seeds are almost as rich as orange juice.

The fruits of some varieties of rose (rose hips) are so rich in vitamin C that they are used in Denmark (and possibly elsewhere) as commercial sources of this vitamin.

Another good fruit, with respect to vitamin C content, is the banana. It is particularly useful in the feeding of babies. In fact, vitamins B and C have rehabilitated the banana in the infant dietary. Not many years ago, if a baby was seen eating a banana, there would be cries of consternation from the onlookers and prophecies of dire consequences. Now, the myth of its indigestibility has vanished along with a good many other dietetic myths. Its value as a source of vitamin B and carbohydrate has already been pointed out (in Chapter V). It is an equally good source of vitamin C. One banana contains about 7 milligrams of vitamin C, more than half the daily requirement of a baby less than a year old.

Vitamin C in Vegetables

For many people, for about a century and a half now, the chief source of vitamin C has been the potato. Uncooked it contains from 35 to 75 milligrams per pound. Much of the vitamin is lost in the cooking if the potatoes are sliced before cooking. To conserve the vitamin the whole potato should be dropped in boiling water and left there for a few minutes. As they are usually cooked (whole), one potato contains about 15 milligrams. White potatoes are richer in vitamin C than sweet potatoes. Fried potatoes contain practically none.

One of the cheapest rich vegetable sources of vitamin C is cabbage. It contains from 100 to 200 milligrams per pound (fresh weight), but the usual method of cooking cabbage results in the destruction of nearly all the vitamin. In order to preserve the vitamin in cabbage, it is necessary to plunge the leaves first into boiling water for a few minutes and then to cook them at a high temperature for as short a time as is necessary to make the cabbage palatable.

Some loss of vitamin C in cooking vegetables is unavoidable; nearly all is lost if the water is discarded or if soda is used. Heating in the presence of air causes a rapid destruction of the vitamin. This destruction is accelerated if copper cooking utensils are used. Heat, air, and soda are even more destructive of this vitamin than they are of vitamin B. Canned vegetables, including the water, contain half or less than half the vitamin C of fresh vegetables.

Freshly cut grass is not ever likely to find a place in human diet. But it is amusing to know that it is possibly the richest of all vegetables in vitamin C. It contains about 350 milligrams per pound. Weight for weight, it is more potent than orange juice. Nebuchadnezzar, whatever his other failings, at least proceeded on a sound dietetic principle.

Brussels sprouts and watercress are almost as rich in vitamin C as grass. It is a pity that watercress is not used instead of head lettuce in salads, for head lettuce contains only negligible quantities of vitamin C.

Dry cereals and pulses—oats, barley, lentils, peas, and beans—are devoid of antiscorbutic potency. After soaking in water and germination for two or three days, however, the sprouts contain significant amounts of the vitamin. Bean sprouts, for example, contain from one-third to two-thirds the vitamin C content of orange juice, weight for weight.

This important fact was rediscovered in 1912. It was known as long ago as 1782. Curtis, reporting in 1807 on the work of Young in the British Navy, wrote:

To be sure, we cannot have a kitchen garden at sea, and a short and scanty crop of greens can only be raised on board ship; but beans and pease and barley and other seeds brought under the malting and vegetating process, are converted into the state of a growing plant . . . and if eaten in this state without any sort of preparation, except that of separating or rejecting the husks, cannot fail to supply what is wanted for the cure of scurvy. . . .

Vitamin C in Milk

The baby nursing at its mother's breast, even up to six months of age, receives adequate amounts of vitamin C in the milk alone; but not after this, or if the mother's diet is low in vitamin C. The bottle-fed baby, on the other hand, requires a vitamin C supplement early. Cow's milk obtained under even the best conditions is an unreliable source of this vitamin. It contains only about one-sixth the vitamin C of human milk.

Although about half the vitamin C of cow's milk is lost in pasteurization, less in modern processes, this does not constitute an argument against the process. At best, cow's milk is a poor source of the vitamin, and the loss in pasteurizing is more than compensated for by the safeguards which the process affords. When a baby is bottle-fed, some vitamin C supplement is necessary; citrus fruit juices and tomato juice should be used.

Most condensed milks retain a considerable portion of their vitamin C; the modern roller-drying process preserves nearly all the vitamin. When it is necessary to boil milk to make it safe, the destruction of its vitamin C can be minimized by bringing the milk to a boil quickly and then boiling it for about three minutes. The saucepan used should contain no trace of copper.

The Tragedy of the Scott South Pole Expedition:
Meat an Inadequate Source of Vitamin C[2]

Fresh meat is frequently referred to as an important anti-scorbutic. Actually it is rather a poor source of vitamin C. It is better than nothing; it may afford some protection in an emergency. But it is not to be relied on for the amounts necessary for abundant health or for strenuous physical activity under adverse conditions. Had this been known in 1911, it might have averted the tragedy of the Scott South Pole Expedition.

In the autumn of 1911 two independent expeditions set out for the South Pole—one, Norwegian, led by Amundsen; the other, English, under Scott. Both started from the edge of the Ross Ice Barrier about 350 miles apart; the distance to the Pole in each case was about 850 miles. Both expeditions had been in camp in the Antarctic for nearly a year. During this time they had put down a number of depots of food and fuel part of the way to the Pole, in order to lighten the loads on the final march.

Amundsen and four companions started on October 20 and arrived at the Pole on December 14, averaging 15½ miles a day. The return was uneventful, averaging 22½ miles a day. The five men and the dogs they had not killed for food arrived at the starting point in excellent condition.

The English expedition began its march on November 1. A party of five arrived at the Pole on January 17, one month

[2] *R. F. Scott*, Scott's Last Expedition, The Personal Journals, *New York, 1913; R. Amundsen*, The South Pole, *New York, 1913.*

later than Amundsen, averaging on the outward journey about 11½ miles a day.

Scott and his party that reached the Pole perished on the return journey at the end of March, only 11 miles (two days' march in their exhausted condition) from food and fuel. They had lost time, with fatal consequences, slowing their pace for two of their five who had broken down. One of these two men died on the march; the other voluntarily left the tent and walked to his death alone in the blizzard in order to save his companions by not holding them back any longer.

It was too late. Scott and his two remaining companions died in their tent during the raging blizzard. After one of the greatest marches in history, 1600 miles on foot (during which they climbed and descended 10,000 feet of glacier) over a desert of snow, they failed with only 11 miles to go to safety.

There were two important and, as it turned out, probably vital, differences between the Norwegian and English expeditions—transport and food. The Norwegians relied entirely on Eskimo dogs, the English on ponies and dogs. The pony transport broke down while the depots of food and fuel were being put down. This misfortune reduced the amount of food and fuel which the Scott expedition could carry.

Regarding his food Amundsen wrote:

It was our aim all through to employ fruit, and vegetables to the greatest possible extent; there is undoubtedly no better means of avoiding sickness. Previously the pemmican had contained nothing but the desired mixture of meat and lard; ours had besides these vegetables and oatmeal.

Their rations on the march consisted of this modified pemmican, dried milk, chocolate, and oatmeal biscuits, "an excellent product consisting of oatmeal, sugar, and dried milk." In addition, they had frozen seal beef and fresh dog meat. "Sweatmeats, jam, fruit, cheese, etc., we had left behind at Framheim the base." They had an abundance of food of high quality.

We may guess at the diet of the English expedition from the following excerpts from Scott's diary:

We are living extraordinarily well at the base. At dinner last night we had some excellent thick seal soup, very much like thick hare soup: this was followed by an equally tasty seal steak and kidney pie and a fruit jelly . . . at breakfast each of us had two of our nutty little Nothemia fish after our bowl of porridge . . . bread and butter and marmalade finished the meal. At the midday meal we had bread and butter, cheese, and cake, and tonight I smell mutton in the preparation. Under the circumstances it would be difficult to conceive more appetizing repasts or a regime which is less likely to produce scorbutic symptoms. I cannot think we shall get scurvy.

Later, on the march, about three weeks from the Pole, Scott wrote the following description of a supper:

We had four courses. The first, pemmican [presumably old style without vegetables], full whack, with slices of horse meat flavored with onion and curry powder and thickened with biscuit; then an arrowroot, cocoa and biscuit hoosh sweetened; then a plum pudding; then cocoa with raisins, and finally a dessert of caramel ginger.

It is clear now that Scott was misled regarding the anti-scorbutic quality of his food. His diet was inferior to Amundsen's also in calcium and probably in vitamin B. During the preceding winter a party of Scott's men made a journey to the rookery of the Emperor penguins. It was probably the worst journey ever survived by human beings. They developed scurvy. One member of Scott's supporting party (who returned before reaching the Pole) came down with scurvy on the return journey. His whole party, after some time on the march, was near the borderline of manifest scurvy. The reason was that the bodily stores of vitamin C (and vitamin B as well) are depleted in a few weeks; and the quality of their diet on the march was not good enough for the tremendous labor of sledge-pulling.

Scott and his men during their return from the Pole lost the ability to heal blisters and frostbite. After that, their stamina ebbed quickly in the bitter weather. It is a reasonable guess that vitamin C deficiency was, in an important measure, responsible for this deterioration, although none of the party developed manifest scurvy. Also, the vitamin B in their diet was inadequate for the exertion of sledge-pulling over a surface that was "like desert sand, not the least slide in the world," for hundreds of miles on the Ross Barrier. Toward the end, the actual amount of food became short. If their diet had been better, if it had supported the stamina of the two failing members of the party a little more, they might all have got in ahead of the fatal blizzard by the necessary two days, to the food and fuel that were waiting for them. This heroic, bitter march would not then have ended in tragedy.

We are not all polar explorers. But the story has its moral for us. Hard physical work calls not only for extra food, but even more for extra vitamins. Amundsen and his men ate rather lightly, but the quality of their diet was excellent. We cannot in good times put down a store of vitamins B and C in our bodies that will last for more than a few weeks. Our diet must provide all these vitamins as we go along;

and "enough" will vary according to the amount of physical work we are doing and the conditions under which we are living.

Crystalline Vitamin C
(Cevitamic Acid, Ascorbic Acid)

Crystalline vitamin C is now quite cheap. In fact, on a basis of economy it can compete with citrus fruits as a source of vitamin C. A palatable drink can be made of crystalline vitamin C dissolved in water, with a little citric acid and sugar added. The crystalline product is probably the cheapest concentrated form of the vitamin; it is certainly the most convenient for expeditions and camping trips. In wartime, under conditions of siege, enough can be flown in to prevent scurvy even in a large city. One pound of vitamin C will prevent scurvy in one hundred adults for three months.

During the siege of Madrid a Spanish friend of the author's tried unavailingly to get permission from the military authorities to have a truckload of oranges brought up to the city from Valencia. Later, when he was telling the story of his failure to get this preventive of scurvy, he was chagrined to learn that a pound of cevitamic acid, which he could have had brought in by plane, would have had the same scurvy-preventing power as a ton of oranges and would certainly have cost no more.

Vitamin C and Resistance to Infection

When the vitamin C in the diet is near or below the minimum necessary for protection against scurvy, health generally is poor and, of course, resistance to infection is subnormal. The practical question, then, regarding resistance to infection is, how common is mild vitamin C deficiency? Analyses of the tissues of people who died in a hospital in an eastern American city indicated that 20 to 30 per cent of these people had too little vitamin C. The percentage was larger still in the older members of this group.

Do these figures indicate that 20 to 30 per cent of adults in the United States are not getting enough vitamin C for good health? There are not enough data to answer this question. The percentage will certainly vary with locality and economic status. A recent analysis of the diets of people in southern California showed that even the poorest obtained an abundance of vitamin C. But citrus fruits and fresh vegetables are relatively cheap and easy to get the year round in southern California. The situation is probably not as good in the large cities in the central and northeastern parts of the United States. Orr's estimates[3] indicate that about 30 per cent of the population of England and Scotland are subsisting on a vitamin C intake below the safe level. As a result, these people very probably offer a lower resistance to infection.

On the other hand, there is no convincing evidence that resistance to infection can be raised much above normal by taking (orally) very large doses of this or any other vitamin.

---

[3] *John Boyd Orr*, Food, Health and Income, *London, 1936, p. 35.*

A recent study with a large number of patients having pulmonary tuberculosis showed an insignificant benefit when these patients were given large quantities of orange juice daily. There are some indications that in cases of gastro-intestinal tuberculosis the benefit from large doses of vitamin C may be significant. In experimental animals the injection of massive doses of vitamin C, corresponding to fifty to seventy times the optimal amount recommended here for human beings, increased several-fold the antibodies (agents combating bacteria) circulating in the blood; but the effect of doses practical for human beings was negligible. It is certain that the administration of massive doses of crystalline vitamin C or great quantities of citrus fruit juices to people who are not ill is simply wasteful as a means of conferring special protection against infection.

Another Antiscorbutic Agent?

One of the clinical tests for latent (early) scurvy is the measurement of the resistance of the capillaries (microscopic blood vessels) in the skin to rupture when the pressure within them is artificially increased by the application of external pressure. In human scurvy the capillary resistance is low. After crystalline vitamin C became available commercially, it was found in many cases that the capillary resistance could not be increased even by administration of large doses of the crystalline vitamin. On the other hand, lemon juice appears to be effective in improving this condition. One group of workers interprets these findings as evidence that there is another vitamin which is also important in the prevention and cure of human scurvy. They do not dispute the necessity

CHAPTER VII

Vitamin D, the Preventive of Rickets

Vitamin D and Rickets

VITAMIN D, which was discovered in 1918, is peculiar among the vitamins in that more of it is ordinarily taken into the body through the skin than by mouth. A deficiency of vitamin D results in rickets. This is a chronic disease of children, occurring between the ages of six months and two years. Although it is rarely if ever fatal, it may cause permanent deformity and other serious after-effects. Dark-skinned children are more prone to it than light-skinned. Thus, in New York City, it was found more frequently and in greater severity among Negro and Italian children.

It was, and probably still is, commoner among the poor than the well-to-do, commoner in overcrowded cities, commoner in climates where there is much rain and fog. Hence, in Continental Europe it is called "the English disease."

Rickets is a disease of the growing parts of the bone in which less than normal amounts of calcium and phosphate are deposited. The fundamental disturbance is actually not in the bones but in the blood itself. Vitamin D governs the amount of calcium and phosphate in the blood; when there is a deficiency of vitamin D, the amount of these necessary materials becomes subnormal. Increasing the intake of calcium and phosphate may do a little good, but the vitamin D intake should also be increased. So while the vitamin has no direct effect on the process of bone formation, without it there cannot be an adequate supply of the necessary bone-forming materials.

In rickets the growing zones become much widened and the bone structure becomes soft. As it softens it is less able to bear normal strains. Since the bones are soft, they are easily deformed. The typical picture of a severely rachitic child is one with a squarish head and protruding bosses on the forehead, bad teeth, a pigeon-breast rather sharp in front with wide flaring ribs, and bowlegs. The pelvis is deformed. Women who have had severe rickets in childhood may in consequence have serious difficulty in child-bearing.

If the disease is cured in early childhood, there are no permanent deformities of the bones. But if it is allowed to go on into late childhood, nothing can be done—the defects are permanent.[1]

Rickets Is Inevitable Unless—

Today more than half the children in the cities of the temperate zones bear some of the stigmata of rickets. The disease is inevitable in the temperate zones unless one of three preventive measures is taken:

1. administration of vitamin D
2. exposure of the naked body to adequate amounts of summer sunlight in the country or at the seashore

---

[1] *Besides being indispensable as an antirachitic, vitamin D is also important in the development of healthy teeth. This is discussed in detail in Chapter IX.*

3. adequate irradiation of the naked body by suitable ultraviolet light

The safest method is the administration of vitamin D.

Human Requirements of Vitamin D

There has been much controversy over the amounts of vitamin D required to prevent and cure rickets. The reasons for this disagreement are the multiplicity of antirachitic substances (seven have been identified); the variation in potency according to the food in which the vitamin is contained; and the need of larger amounts to cure the disease than to prevent it.

An adequate curative dose of vitamin D is 3000 units (International or U. S. P. XI Units) daily. But when rickets is actually present, its treatment should never be undertaken by an untrained person.

The more important problem for the layman is the prevention of rickets. Taken in the form of "vitamin D" milk, which we shall discuss in more detail later, 400 units of vitamin D daily are an adequate preventive. But in addition, the vitamin D intake should provide for a good rate of growth and healthy teeth. For this purpose larger doses are necessary: infants two to three weeks old should have 350 units daily; during the second month, 700 units daily; later and until puberty, 1000 units daily. High grade cod- or halibut-liver oil contains about 375 units in a teaspoonful. Even with these doses of cod-liver oil (or vitamin D in other forms), a child of school age should receive a quart of whole milk daily.

Nothing is known regarding the vitamin D requirement of grown people. Although there has been no experimental or clinical demonstration that they require this vitamin, it seems likely that they do need some. Vitamin D assists in the maintenance of the proper amounts of calcium and phosphate in the blood; these are required by adults as well as children for many purposes, among others for the reconstruction of bone, which is a living tissue constantly undergoing wear and tear. One can only guess the vitamin D requirement for adults for this purpose. Our guess is that about 200 units daily—the amount in a pint of "vitamin D" milk—may be enough.

Vitamin D Requirement of Expectant and Nursing Mothers

There is no question that expectant and nursing mothers require vitamin D. Adequate amounts of this vitamin and of calcium and phosphate are necessary for the proper development of the bones and teeth in the child before it is born and for the protection of the mother's teeth.

A woman who is nursing a child requires vitamin D to assist her body in retaining the calcium and phosphate from her food. A large amount of these minerals passes into her milk. When she does not obtain and retain enough from her food, her bones and teeth give up their calcium and phosphate to the milk.

Expectant and nursing mothers, therefore, require a quart of milk daily, preferably "vitamin D" milk, plus a vitamin D supplement of 1000 to 2000 units daily, but not more. This supplement need not be obtained entirely from the drug store. In the summer months in the Southern states and in California a considerable amount can be obtained by reasonable sun-bathing during the late morning.

Sources of Vitamin D

None of the foods is a good source of vitamin D. Only egg-yolk, milk, and butter contain more than negligible amounts, and these cannot furnish the total amount required daily. One is driven, therefore, to the use of special vitamin D preparations. Of these there are three main types. One contains a substance called ergosterol which has been converted to the vitamin by suitable irradiation (i.e., exposure to ultraviolet light) and subsequently more or less purified. This so-called activated ergosterol is suspended in some oil, usually corn oil. The dose is in drops and is generally printed on the label. But this form of vitamin D should not be used except under the direction of a physician.

A new development in the preparation of ergosterol concentrates promises to be useful. It has been reported that a single injection of a large dose of pure vitamin D will prevent rickets for a whole winter. The dose used was 15 milligrams (about 1/2000 of an ounce) suspended in a little oil. Ten times this amount taken by mouth was ineffective. This method may prove to be particularly useful in institutions and schools. There the labor of daily administration of drops or teaspoonfuls of oil taken by mouth throughout the autumn and winter could be replaced by one injection which could be given to a whole school on a single day.

Another vehicle of vitamin D is one of the refined fish-liver oils. Cod-liver oil was the old standby, but it has been super-seded by other, more potent fish-liver oils such as halibut. The dosage is in teaspoonfuls or tablespoonfuls. One reason for preferring this variety to ergosterol preparations is that it is also rich in vitamin A. Another reason, to be discussed later, is that there is less danger of overdosage.

The third rich source is "vitamin D" milk, of which there are two kinds, equally good. In one the vitamin content is increased to 430 units per quart by direct ultraviolet ir-radiation of the milk. This is "fortified vitamin D milk." The other form, "metabolized vitamin D milk," is obtained by feeding the cows yeast which has been irradiated with ultraviolet light. Part of the vitamin D so formed passes from the yeast into the milk. "Metabolized vitamin D milk" is also standardized to contain 430 units per quart. Since milk is a good source of calcium and phosphate, the special value of "vitamin D" milk is that the vitamin and the materials upon which it acts are taken together. But for chil-dren even a daily quart of "vitamin D" milk will not supply the desirable amount of the vitamin. Hence, a supplement such as one of the fish-liver oils should be taken also.

Antirachitic Value of Milk: Calcium and Phosphate

An adequate intake of physiologically available calcium and phosphate is as necessary as vitamin D. Children re-quire until puberty about one gram of calcium and some-what more phosphate daily. The adult requirement is about 0.7 gram of calcium and about 1.3 grams of phosphorus daily. This can be supplied by milk. Children who do not drink their daily quart of milk, and nearly all adults, have a diet deficient in calcium and phosphate.

Vitamin D Overdosage

Of all the vitamins, vitamin D is the only one with which at present there is danger of harmful overdosage. The symptoms of acute overdosage are increased frequency of urination, loss of appetite, nausea, vomiting, diarrhoea, muscular weakness, lassitude, and dizziness. These symptoms quickly disappear when the overdosage is stopped. The effects of overdosage for a long period are deposits of calcium where normally no such deposits occur—for example, in the kidneys and blood vessels.

Babies are more sensitive than older children or adults. Except in a very rare case there is no danger whatever in the doses recommended above. Larger doses should not be taken save under close observation by a physician. Exposure of a naked baby for long periods to strong sunlight, or to ultraviolet light, is not to be recommended because the amount of vitamin D so obtained is uncertain. Ergosterol concentrates, of which the dose is in drops, are dangerous in the hands of a zealous but inadequately instructed mother. But there is no risk with the fish-liver oils or "vitamin D" milks.

The Prevention of Rickets by Sunlight

An interesting scientific problem arose when it was discovered that rickets could be cured by two quite different methods, by a substance—vitamin D—and by sunlight and ultraviolet light.

For a few years the mystically inclined enjoyed themselves with this apparent demonstration of the equivalence of Matter and Energy for Life. The game did not last long. The problem was soon solved, and the answer was simple. A specific part of the ultraviolet rays in the sunlight is able to convert certain substances present in some foods and in the skin into another form, which then has the property of curing and preventing rickets. The process of conversion is called "activation." Before these substances are activated they are called provitamins; seven of them are now known. They possess no antirachitic properties unless and until they are activated. The chemical change in the provitamin during the activation process is a very simple one, and activation of provitamins in food materials by ultraviolet light is now a large industry.

When the skin is exposed to sunlight or ultraviolet light, activation of a provitamin in the skin occurs. This provitamin is probably synthesized in the animal body; there is also some in the food. Whatever its origin, it is carried into the skin by the blood. After activation in the skin by sunlight or ultraviolet light, the vitamin is transported by the blood all over the body. Hence the antirachitic effect of sunlight and ultraviolet light.

The antirachitic potency of sunlight is restricted to a certain small fraction of its ultraviolet rays.[2] The antirachitic part of the sunlight which penetrates to the earth's surface

---

[2] *The quality of radiation is measured in wave lengths, whether it is visible light or invisible infrared and ultraviolet rays. The unit of length here is called the angstrom unit, for which the symbol is Å.*

lies between 3130 Å and 2900 Å. The rays at 3130 Å are about one hundred times less effective than those near 2950 Å.

The limitation of sunlight as an antirachitic agent is that except in the summer, and even then only on clear days, very little of the antirachitic portion of the light penetrates to the earth's surface. Thus in Chicago in December the shortest wave length to penetrate is near 3050 Å; in May it is 2990 Å; and in summer, 2900 Å. Since the main antirachitic portion lies between 3000 Å and 2900 Å, there is practically no antirachitic potency even in bright sunlight in late autumn, winter, and spring. The figures obtained in Chicago probably hold for the whole of the temperate zone.

Rain, dust, fog, and smoke reduce to almost zero the amount of antirachitic sunlight which penetrates to the earth's surface. For this reason the best time for sun-bathing is between 10 and 11 o'clock in the morning.

The ultraviolet radiation will penetrate one layer of light summer clothing. When the skin is heavily tanned, less of the ultraviolet light reaches the lower layer of the skin where it activates the provitamin. This is the reason for the greater incidence of rickets in dark-skinned children. This is also an argument against developing a heavy coat of tan. It may cause admiration among one's friends, but it decreases the scientific profit from exposure to sunshine.

The ultraviolet light from sun-lamps is, of course, as effective as sunlight when the lamps produce light of suitable wave length. The difficulty with such lamps is that they deteriorate, and the wave length of the light emitted changes. Unless they are checked periodically they should not be relied on to cure or prevent rickets.

Sunlight Alone Cannot Prevent Rickets

The effectiveness of sunlight alone as an antirachitic agent is one of the important questions involved in preventing rickets in a whole population. In order to get reliable evidence on this point, an investigation was recently made in two Pacific Coast cities, Portland, Oregon, and San Diego, California. Portland has an average of 2194 hours of sunshine per year; San Diego is better off by 38 per cent, with 3024 hours. In Portland during the winter the sun may not appear for days at a time; the winter climate of San Diego is sunny and mild.

In each of these two cities a large number of five-year-old children coming from all social classes in fairly representative cross-section were examined for rickets. In Portland 95 per cent, in San Diego 73 per cent of the children had four or more signs of rickets. We must conclude, then, that with our present mode of life even abundant sunshine as in San Diego does not furnish adequate protection against rickets.

In both cities most of the children had received some antirachitic medication (83 per cent in Portland, 82 per cent in San Diego). The amount and regularity of the medication and the persistence in its use had obviously been inadequate. Most children after the age of two or three are no longer under the observation of a doctor, and consequently their diet gradually deteriorates toward that of their parents.

Similar figures for the prevalence of rickets could probably be obtained all through the temperate zone. For instance, in the English cities of Manchester, Birmingham, and London, when large groups of children were examined, 85 per cent of all of them were found to have one or more signs of rickets.

Such figures show the need on the part of the health authorities for an intensive and constant educational campaign against rickets. The disease is easily prevented. There are effective antirachitic activities for every purse and palate—the fish-liver oils, "vitamin D" milk, vitamin D concentrates. Effective ultraviolet lamps could be installed in the schools at relatively little expense and operated by the school nurses.

Children are not the least of our national resources. Surely it is worth a little extra care and effort—even the spending of public funds—to safeguard them from the physical handicaps in later life which otherwise will inevitably result from rickets.

Cosmetics and the "Sunshine Vitamin"

Recently, through its inclusion in cosmetics, face creams, and soap, vitamin D has come into national advertising. In some cases the advertisements state explicitly, in others the reader is led to believe, that vitamin D enhances the value of the product as a cosmetic. It seems hardly necessary to point out that there is no scientific evidence in support of this claim—and that is putting the matter mildly.

It is true that one recent report of an experiment stated that the metabolism of the skin of vitamin D deficient animals was about 60 per cent that of normal animals, and that the metabolism became normal when adequate amounts of the vitamin were given. But these experimental animals were already severely deficient in the vitamin. And though their skin metabolism was restored to normal, the report does not mention any increase in the beauty of the skin itself.

Perhaps the investigators were not interested in that aspect of the situation. But for anyone buying a cosmetic, that is the one important consideration; and at present there is no evidence that a large amount of vitamin D taken by a normal animal—whether human or other—makes any difference in the skin.

Another reason for skepticism is the fact that these advertisements do not state the amount of vitamin D in the preparations they ballyhoo. As nobody knows what the vitamin D requirement of adults is anyway, it is impossible to estimate how much of the vitamin must be put into the face cream, or how many jars of the face cream must be rubbed in daily to make its contribution at all significant. It is highly improbable that the vitamin D intake is materially raised by the amount which is absorbed through the skin from such a "vitamin D face cream." There is, further, no reason to believe that vitamin D rubbed into the skin is any more effective than taken by mouth. It would probably be just as good and a great deal simpler to use the advertised produce as a spread for bread. (And the results, as far as enhancement of beauty is concerned, would be no different.)

The practice of putting vitamin D into soap—the advertisements refer to it as "the sunshine vitamin"—is even more absurd, because we do not customarily leave soap on our faces and bodies long enough for any of the vitamin to be absorbed.

Recently an advertisement appeared recommending a product because it contained provitamin D. At best, this is ignorance trading on credulity, for a provitamin is not a vitamin at all, but a substance that must undergo a chemical change in order to become a vitamin. In this instance the provitamin is presumably ergosterol. It is pointless to take ergosterol in this form, since we already have an abundance of it in our bodies and circulating in the blood. We cannot avoid taking it in our food; the difficulty is in getting it converted into the vitamin. In this respect the advertised provitamin is no better than the provitamin we eat, or than that which is made in the body.

It will repay the prospective customer here especially to ask: How much of the vitamin is there in this advertised product? How much does it cost per unit of vitamin? Can it be obtained more cheaply and more effectively in some other form?

CHAPTER VIII

Vitamins E, F, and K: Birth, Beauty, and Death

§1

Vitamin E, Misnamed the "Antisterility Vitamin"

VITAMIN E is necessary for reproduction in animals; it is required by both the male and the female. Nevertheless, its popular name, the "antisterility vitamin," is almost completely misleading.

Severe vitamin E deficiency in men irreparably damages the tissues in the testes which produce the sperm. No amount of vitamin E therapy can then repair the damage. Therefore such men become permanently sterile. To the extent, then, that a sufficient vitamin E intake prevents this damage from occurring, it may accurately be called the "antisterility vitamin," but beyond this the phrase is a misnomer.

A woman who is severely deficient in vitamin E cannot carry a pregnancy through successfully. She has an early miscarriage. But after being fed vitamin E, she has no difficulty with a subsequent pregnancy. In a woman, therefore, the harm done by a vitamin E deficiency is not permanent. She is not sterile. Sterility is a condition in which, for one reason or another, the ovum (egg) is not fertilized; in other words, there is a failure of conception. A woman deficient in vitamin E is not sterile, for she can become pregnant. Her difficulty is in carrying a pregnancy through successfully. Since vitamin E corrects this condition, it would be more accurate to call it the "antimiscarriage vitamin."

Sources of Vitamin E

The richest source of vitamin E is wheat-germ oil. In wheat and corn all the vitamin E is in the embryo of the grain; there is none in the endosperm (the part that forms the bulk of flour). The oil is formed simply by cold-pressing the germ. It is produced commercially and sold in drug stores. Other vegetable oils such as corn oil and cottonseed oil also contain vitamin E. When any of these vegetable oils become rancid the vitamin is usually destroyed. Cod-liver oil contains no vitamin E.

The leafy green vegetables—lettuce, spinach, and watercress—have an abundance of vitamin E.

The chemical composition of the vitamin has been established in the past few years; it has been synthesized in the laboratory; and it is now in process of commercial manufacture.

How Vitamin E Prevents Miscarriage

An interesting explanation has been proposed of the way in which vitamin E prevents miscarriage. After the ovum has been fertilized by the sperm, it implants itself on the in-side wall of the uterus and thus is enabled to obtain from the maternal blood the nourishment necessary for its development. In this process of attachment a thick pad of tissue—the placenta—is developed. On one side of the placenta is the umbilical cord, which passes from the umbilicus (navel) of the fetus (as the ovum is then called) to the placenta. The cord is simply a fleshy cable containing an artery and a vein for carrying blood to and fro between the fetus and the placenta. The other side of the placenta rests in a lake of blood which it has produced by partly digesting away the adjacent uterine wall.

What keeps the placenta from eating all the way through the uterine wall? The answer lies in one of those marvelous mechanisms of balance which nature manages somehow to contrive. It appears that the placenta itself manufactures a substance which counteracts to some extent the digestive ferments that eat away the uterine wall. The placenta also manufactures the digestive ferments.

In a successful pregnancy a balance is established between the eroding ferments on the one hand and the counteracting substance on the other. The placenta eats its way into the uterine wall deeply enough to get a firm hold and an ample blood supply for the fetus, but not so deeply that it perforates the wall, which would be disastrous.

Some women fail to establish such a successful balance. The placenta manufactures too much of the counteracting substance, with the result that it never develops a firm hold and it eventually loses the tenuous hold it has managed to establish. When this happens there is a spontaneous miscarriage.

The effect of vitamin E, according to the proposed explanation, is to re-establish the balance. It does this by neutralizing the counteracting substance sufficiently to let the digestive ferments of the placenta eat their way into the uterine wall deeply enough so that the placenta will not become loose or separate from the wall prematurely.

Vitamin E in Practice

Experience has shown that while vitamin E therapy is not infallible in preventing spontaneous miscarriage, it can be depended on for a reasonable degree of success. One recent study is indicative of the general results. Three groups of women were studied. The first group consisted of thirty-five women who had previously had two or more spontaneous miscarriages. Each was given a daily dose of one-half teaspoonful of wheat-germ oil, and as a result twenty-five of them were able to carry a pregnancy through successfully. In the second group, of eleven women, each had already had one spontaneous miscarriage. They were given the same daily dose of wheat-germ oil, and nine of the eleven successfully completed a pregnancy. The third group consisted of nineteen women who were threatened with miscarriage in the first three months of pregnancy. For them the daily dose of wheat-germ oil was increased to one tablespoonful; for thirteen of them the pregnancy was successfully carried through.

In the same study a fourth group was used to test the antisterility possibilities of vitamin E. The fifteen women in this group, all sterile, were given a tablespoonful of wheat-germ oil daily, but the treatment did not produce a single successful result.

This study and others which have obtained similar results justify the description of vitamin E as the antimiscarriage rather than the antisterility vitamin.

Such massive doses as those described above are not required, it should be emphasized, by the great majority of pregnant women. For them the amounts of vitamin E in the leafy vegetables eaten daily are sufficient. Wheat-germ oil is required only by women who have a tendency to spontaneous miscarriage, and even then it should be taken only under the direction of a physician.

The explanation of the action of vitamin E given above shows that the vitamin is required only in cases where a salutary balance has not been established and there has consequently been a pathological failure of the placenta to implant itself firmly in the uterine wall. If too much vitamin E is taken—and this may well occur in a normal woman taking large amounts of wheat-germ oil—the placenta may become so firmly imbedded that after the child is born the uterus may have difficulty in casting the placenta off; so far there have been no reports of the placenta eating through the wall.

Vitamin E and Certain Spinal Diseases

Chronic vitamin E deficiency in animals produces a weakening and shrinkage of the muscles, accompanied by degeneration in the spinal cord. The pathological picture of the animal resembles certain rather rare human diseases which have been hitherto incurable. In one of these (amyotrophic lateral sclerosis), treatment with very large doses of vitamin E has brought encouraging results, especially in young people.

§2

"Vitamin F," the "Skin Vitamin"

Women's magazines for some months carried large advertisements of "vitamin F," the "skin vitamin." These advertisements referred, with illustrations, to experimental work which demonstrated the necessity in the diet of two substances. These were not named, but from the general description the advertisers obviously meant linoleic and linolenic acids. A dietary deficiency of these acids is very difficult to produce experimentally because they are found in nearly all foods, and the amounts required are easily supplied by the ordinary diet. Experimental work on rats has produced no evidence that the skin is especially benefited by these substances. In fact, the obvious sign of deficiency is in the tail! While this may be a matter of grave concern for the rats, it can hardly agitate human beings very profoundly.

There are no data regarding the human requirement of "vitamin F." From the amount required by the rat we may guess that the total daily requirement of human adults is supplied by two tablespoonfuls of corn oil, which is common salad dressing. Even without the corn oil there are very probably adequate amounts in the ordinary diet. Olive oil and egg-yolk contain some, but rather less, of these two acids than corn oil does. Tung oil, poppyseed, and linseed oil are very rich sources. There is no "vitamin F" in butter.

"Vitamin F face creams," which are advertised to "make you beautiful while you sleep," probably do not contain more "vitamin F" per jar than do two teaspoonfuls of salad oil.

Nutritional science is in no position to pass on the value of such preparations as aids to beauty, though it may have its doubts. At any rate, "vitamin F" applied externally is certainly no more effective than when taken by mouth; and getting the vitamin by smearing oneself with face cream is a bothersome and expensive means of securing a negligible amount.

The Prevention of Death from Hemorrhage: Vitamin K and the Clotting of Blood

The phenomenon of the clotting of the blood has been studied by physiologists for more than a century. If the blood did not clot in a wound, a scratch would cause fatal hemorrhage, childbirth would always be fatal for the mother, and surgery would be impossible.

An investigation into an artificial hemorrhagic disease of fowl discovered a substance which has turned out to be useful in human surgery because it accelerates the abnormally slow clotting of blood in certain conditions. This substance is called vitamin K.

The hemorrhagic disease in birds is the result of a diminished ability of the blood to clot. The immediate cause of this deficiency is a diminution of a substance in the blood which is essential for the clotting process in all animals. This essential substance is called prothrombin. When chicks are maintained on a diet deficient in vitamin K for fourteen to twenty-four days, the amount of prothrombin in the blood is reduced to a pathologically low level. Restoration of vitamin K to the diet is followed by an increase in the prothrombin in the blood, and the hemorrhagic disease is cured. Vitamin K and prothrombin are different substances, but the amount of the vitamin apparently determines the amount of pro-thrombin.

Human beings and other animals—rats, guinea pigs, and young dogs—can dispense with vitamin K in the diet. In them it is synthesized by bacteria in the intestine, whence it is absorbed by the blood and lymph. The vitamin is fat-soluble; when there is interference with the normal mechanism for the absorption of fat from the intestine into the body, the absorption of vitamin K, even in animals other than birds, is also retarded.

In human beings this difficulty arises when there is lack of bile in the intestine. This occurs, for example, when the bile duct from the gall-bladder or liver is obstructed by a stone in the duct, or by cancer. The bile duct from the gall-bladder empties into the intestine. The bile which it delivers is essential for the absorption of fats, carotenoids, and vitamin K. When bile is absent from the intestine these substances are not absorbed.

One of the dangers in surgical operations to relieve obstruction of the bile duct—these patients are deeply jaundiced—is post-operative hemorrhage, because of the slow clotting of the blood. In the few cases in which it has been tried, the injection of a vitamin K concentrate hastened the clotting of the blood. An extract of alfalfa (alfalfa is rich in vitamin K) mixed with bile (in order to permit the vitamin to be absorbed) taken by mouth achieved the same result. The administration of vitamin K promises, then, to be a useful pre-operative measure in cases of obstructive jaundice.

There is no reason for expecting that vitamin K therapy

will be of any value in hemorrhagic diseases such as hemophilia (a hereditary tendency to profuse bleeding, even from very slight wounds).

Foods rich in vitamin K are green leaves, spinach, alfalfa, and green cabbage. Cereals, wheat-germ oil, carrots, and yeast are poor sources. There is practically none in potatoes, lemon juice, and cod-liver oil.

The chemical constitution of vitamin K is established. In the course of these chemical studies a number of substances which do not occur in foodstuffs were found with vitamin K activity. These substances are, of course, closely related to the naturally occurring vitamin.

Vitamin K is now manufactured commercially. Thus the medical profession can administer vitamin K in massive doses as a safeguard when necessary, and when it is needed quickly in an emergency.

CHAPTER IX

Diet and Dental Health

An Old Story

DENTAL caries (decay) has been one of the afflictions of the human race since time immemorial. There is no need of going into its history in detail, for the evidence is simply iteration of the same fact—that dental decay has always been prevalent. One description of Englishwomen at the end of the sixteenth century may be taken as reasonably typical of the sort of data which we should encounter:

We are sorry to state that one essential of perfect beauty was sorely wanting among these zealous cultivators of their charms— their teeth, instead of being pearly white, were in general black and rotten—and this grievous defect was supposed by foreigners to be occasioned by the inordinate love of the English ladies for sugar. Perhaps to this their love of tobacco might have been added, for many of them were greatly addicted to smoking.[1]

Today we are a little better off than these ladies of an older time. We have been taught to keep our teeth clean (though there is still considerable dispute over the value of tooth-brushing in preventing dental decay); we have been taught to make periodic visits to the dentist, so that decay can be spotted before it has proceeded very far; and modern

---

[1] *Craik and MacFarlane*, The Pictorial History of England, *vol. II, p. 887.*

dental science has developed effective techniques for salvaging teeth in which decay has begun.

But are we much better off so far as the prevalence of decay itself is concerned? On this point the final report of the British Medical Research Council on *The Influence of Diet on Caries in Children's Teeth* (1936) comes to a pessimistic conclusion:

> *The fact that dental disease is still so common, especially among civilized peoples, implies that there is still much to be learned; for there are more dental clinics, many more people brush their teeth, and much more dental treatment is practiced today than ever in the world before. The scourge thereby does not appear to be prevented, in fact it seems to be as prevalent today as it has ever been.*

We might have to resign ourselves to an indefinite continuance of this affliction if it were not that modern nutritional science, and vitamin research especially, provide us with the first really useful clues as to the cause of dental caries and the means of preventing it.

Diet and Dental Health Among Native Peoples

In our second chapter we referred to an investigation among neighboring tribes in East Africa which pointed to a close relationship between diet and dental health. A world survey of this relationship was made by Weston Price. He reached two important conclusions: first, no groups have yet been found building strong bodies and maintaining good health who live on plant foods alone; second, in addition to a liberal source of minerals, all groups successful in maintaining a high immunity to dental caries use some special animal products of high quality which supply the fat-soluble vitamins (A and D).

These conclusions were later confirmed by other independent studies in New Guinea, South America, and the Arctic.

Diet and the Dental Health of Children

In England from 1918 on, Mrs. M. Mellanby began and inspired a series of investigations into the effect of diet on the dental health of children. She was the first to emphasize the importance of vitamin D. In the course of these studies the diet of the children was carefully supervised so that improvements in the caries situation could not be attributed to any cause but the vitamin D supplement. On analysis of the results, the British Medical Research Council reported the following conclusions:

1. A diet high in vitamin D can do much to prevent the occurrence of decay if the vitamin is given while the teeth are developing.

2. A beneficial effect may result if the vitamin is given at a fairly late stage of the development of the teeth.

3. Even if the vitamin is given after the teeth have cut through the gums, the onset and spread of caries may be delayed.

The average age of the children involved in these studies was over ten years. The vitamin D treatment decreased dental decay. The obvious question then was: If the vitamin D had been given at an earlier age (that is, in an earlier stage of the development of the teeth), would the occurrence of dental caries have been less?

This question was answered in a thorough, carefully controlled investigation carried out in Toronto in 1932.[2] Children in two orphanages were selected for this investigation. The diet contained a good supply of milk, meat, eggs, vegetables, and fruit. Throughout the year the children spent a considerable amount of time each day outdoors. They brushed their teeth twice daily. The excellence of the diet and general care of these children is attested to by the fact that without additional vitamin D they averaged 1.5 new cavities in their teeth per child per year, whereas the average for schoolchildren in Toronto was 3.0 cavities per child per year. The ages of the children studied ranged from two to sixteen years.

Each orphanage was divided into two groups: one, the control group, continued the regular diet: the second received exactly the same diet with the addition of eight drops of viosterol (about 1000 units). The vitamin D was incorporated in a plain ginger cooky. The control group received the same cooky with the vitamin D omitted. The only variable factor in the two groups was the administration of vitamin D in the second group.

The method of dental examination was extraordinarily thorough. Casts of the mouth were made at the beginning and at the end of the one-year dietary period. The presence and size of cavities were determined by X-rays as well as by mirror and probe.

---

[2] *By P. G. Anderson, C. H. M. Williams, H. Halderson, C. Summerfeldt, and R. Gordon Agnew.*

Type of Teeth	Age	Group	Average Number of New Cavities per Tooth
Permanent teeth	3–10	vitamin D no vitamin D supplement	0.009 0.050
	11–16	vitamin D no vitamin D supplement	0.041 0.061
Temporary teeth	3–10	vitamin D no vitamin D supplement	0.034 0.100
	11–16	vitamin D no vitamin D supplement	0.037 0.032

The answer is clear. Vitamin D had a marked effect in preventing new-cavity formation in the children of three to ten, and practically no effect in the older children.

For the prevention of both rickets and dental decay the diet must contain, in addition to vitamin D, an adequate amount of calcium and phosphate. These two minerals must be present in approximately equal amounts. This is easiest and best supplied in the form of milk. The advantage of "vitamin D" milk is that in it the vitamin D and these minerals are obtained at the same time. If the calcium in the diet is greatly in excess of the phosphate, more vitamin D is required.

An Easy Way to Protect the Teeth

Before the Toronto investigation, and independent of the English studies, similar observations were made by two American workers, Boyd and Drain, who noticed the effect of a special diet on dental caries. Twenty-eight children admitted to hospitalization for diabetes all had active dental caries. After some time on the strict diabetic diet of the hospital, the dental decay was arrested. Boyd and Drain then tried this dietary regime on children who were not suffering from diabetes. The results were the same: in each case, pre-existing decay was completely arrested in ten weeks.

The important items in the daily diet that Boyd and Drain prescribed were one quart of milk, one egg, two large servings of vegetables, six teaspoonfuls of butter, and one teaspoonful of cod-liver oil. This diet can now be improved by the substitution of "vitamin D" milk for ordinary milk, and also by increasing the dose of cod-liver oil to two teaspoonfuls daily. The items in this diet are, of course, not enough for a day's food, especially for an older child. They can be supplemented by meat, cereals, bread, etc. Children receiving the items above can eat considerable quantities of sweet and starchy foods without hindering the arrest and prevention of tooth decay.

This diet has been used in children's clinics and orphanages in a number of American cities, with the same beneficial effects on dental health.

Another School of Thought

One group of American workers holds views regarding the relation of diet to dental health somewhat different from those presented above. They maintain that there is no relation between the intake of calcium, phosphate, and vitamin D and the incidence of dental decay. They agree that the nature of the diet is important but they hold that the important factor is the amount of sugar. The greater the amount of sugar, the greater the likelihood of dental decay. Bacteria in the mouth, which thrive on the sugar residues left there after a meal, produce acids which erode the enamel and thus expose the inner dentine to bacterial invasion and decay. By reducing the sugar to a minimum, they claim to have reduced significantly the occurrence of dental decay among people whose diet was low in calcium, phosphate, and vitamin D. The only constant difference which they found between the mouths of individuals who had little dental decay and those who had considerable was that the latter harbored more bacteria of the acidophilous groups.

The weight of the evidence found by other workers is overwhelmingly against this view. Every important item of evidence presented in opposition to the significance of calcium, phosphate, and vitamin D in the diet has failed to be confirmed by other workers.

Nevertheless, practically the same diet would be acceptable to either of these two schools of thought. A diet containing milk, eggs, vegetables, and fruit automatically contains little sugar. The cod-liver oil or vitamin D recommended by Boyd and Drain and numerous other American, English, and Canadian workers is certainly necessary for the prevention of rickets. Milk, eggs, vegetables, and fruit are to be recommended also because they provide vitamins A, the B complex, and C, and protein of high biological value.

The Lesson to Be Learned

The bulk of the clinical and experimental work shows that the same dietary factors that determine the original structure of the teeth and bones as they develop also determine the

ability of the teeth to resist infection later in life. When the
dietary conditions are favorable for the development of
sound teeth, these teeth in later life are less susceptible to
decay. On the other hand, when the diet is a poor one as far
as the development of the teeth is concerned, surface injury
is not met by a vigorous recuperative reaction in such teeth.
Bacterial erosion is not resisted, and cavities result.

There can be no doubt, then, regarding the lesson to be
learned from all this. To provide for good dental health,
calcium, phosphate, and vitamins A and D should be eaten
in abundant amounts as early as possible by the pregnant
woman because the teeth begin to develop before the child
is born. The vitamin D especially should be continued during
the time when most of the teeth are formed—that is, until
adolescence.

The Toronto investigators, some of whose results we have
already presented, pointed out:

*It is not generally recognized that a good ordinary diet, containing
adequate amounts of milk, meat, eggs, vegetables, and fruit, is still
deficient in . . . vitamin D. This vitamin is not present in perceptible amounts in fruits and vegetables. The only ordinary foods
that contain it are egg-yolks, and to a slight extent, summer milk and
summer butter. It requires approximately 5 egg-yolks to furnish the
vitamin D equivalent of one teaspoonful of cod-liver oil. . . . . Fish
oils are, of course, an excellent source of this vitamin, and their use
is now universal [?] with small infants and children for the prevention of rickets; but owing to their rather disagreeable taste, and
a lack of appreciation of a need of them, they are generally not
consumed by the older child or adult.*

The Vitamin D Requirement for Dental Health

A recently published study indicates that in order to prevent or retard tooth decay a child needs about 1000 units of vitamin D daily. This is twice to four times the minimum amount required for the prevention of rickets. This difference accounts for the fact that dental caries is more prevalent than rickets in children, and for the frequent observation that the presence or absence of rickets and the occurrence of dental decay do not run parallel. Even when no correlation was found between rickets and the incidence of dental decay, it was observed that children with a history of rickets had more malocclusion (misfit between the grinding surfaces of the upper and lower teeth).

And So What?

Vitamin D was discovered in 1918. The wife of the discoverer, Mrs. Mellanby, demonstrated in the succeeding ten years by experiments on animals and observations on children the importance of this vitamin for dental health. Boyd and Drain published their observations in 1929. The work of the Toronto investigators and others was published by 1934. Yet "the scourge of dental disease . . . is as prevalent today as it has ever been." This is not because the knowledge and the means of preventing it are lacking; it is because the knowledge has not yet got into wide enough circulation.

What Hope Is There for the Teeth of Adults?

After puberty the beneficial effects of liberal amounts of vitamins on the teeth are small. Nevertheless, it is unlikely that the last word has yet been said on this subject so far as adults are concerned. How many adults obtain a diet really abundant in all the vitamins, calcium, and phosphate?

CHAPTER X

Diets for Children and Adults

IT WOULD be fatuous to expect any adult who thinks he is healthy to follow for long any dietary instructions, unless for reducing. But children, even in this day and age are under their mothers' control at least for their meals. What seemed simpler, then, than to draw up a list of twenty-one meals incorporating all the lore and advice in the foregoing chapters? At least the children would benefit.

The author accordingly consulted dietitians and prepared a list of twenty-one meals for children. Then at the thought of proposing them to his own nine-year-old daughter, he cringed and his crusading ardor failed. The twenty-one meals went into the wastepaper basket. It was more realistic to draw up general directions that leave much latitude for individual taste and circumstances.

A Diet for Children

Every child should receive daily one quart of milk (preferably "vitamin D" milk), one egg, two large servings of fresh leafy vegetables, six teaspoonfuls of butter, and a tall glass of citrus fruit or tomato juice. Some of the milk may be incorporated into soups, puddings, and custard. The egg is best well boiled, for three to five minutes, or it may be disguised by addition to something else. It should not be fried.

This will not supply enough vitamin D. If the child does not object to the taste of the prepared fish-liver oils these are the cheapest form in which additional vitamins A and D can be given, about two teaspoonfuls daily. If the child dislikes the fish-liver oils, vitamin A and D capsules can be bought. One of these daily will be enough. Or viosterol can be used. The dose is eight to fifteen drops. It is tasteless and mixes with milk or almost any other food. The vitamin D supplement should be continued until adolescence.

Some rich source of the vitamin B complex must be supplied. The cheapest form is the cereal, "the scalp of the sizings," described in the chapter on vitamin B (Chapter V). This can be prepared like any other cooked cereal. Since children tire of cooked cereals when served day in and day out, for variety this cereal can be made up into muffins, pancakes, tea biscuits, even bread.

If this or similar cereal (with approximately the same vitamin B content) is not available or is unacceptable, the only alternatives are dried brewer's yeast and the rather expensive liquid B concentrates.

Enough of the cereal or other vitamin B supplement should be eaten to supply daily at least 10 International Units of thiamine (vitamin B_1) per pound of body weight.

Other cereals, oatmeal and cornmeal will supply calories and some protein, but they are not as good sources of vitamin B. Farina containing wheat germ is a good source of vitamin B, but it is not readily obtainable.

Meat should (the word "should" is invidious but it is hard to avoid) be on the menu at least three times a week. There is no reason against serving it once every day. For most nutritional purposes beef, veal, lamb, mutton, lean pork, and fowl are alike. Fried meat cannot be recommended. Fried bacon should not be used to replace other meat.

After these essentials have been attended to, everything else can be left to habits, taste, purse, and appetite. Additional calories will be supplied by potatoes, bread, crackers, and the desserts. Relatively little bread is eaten in the United States; commercial whole-wheat bread in preference to white bread is worth fighting for only where a good deal of bread is eaten.

Watercress, romaine lettuce, other leafy greens, and parsley are more nutritious than head lettuce in green salads.

The child's weight is a sufficient guide to the amount it should be eating. A child of thirteen requires as much food as an adult. If the appetite is poor, the mother would be well advised to study the tables on pages 167 and 168 and attend to her cooking instead of badgering the child, before she consults a physician.

There is no reason for prohibiting reasonable amounts of candy, cake, pie, and ice cream, so long as they are not eaten when they would spoil the appetite for the next meal. Too many desserts consist of stewed fruit, custard, and the stodgy puddings beloved of dietitians. One does not eat for vitamins alone. There is physiological evidence that unpleasant meals, regardless of what the food is, are bad meals. But the dictum that eating should be a pleasure, even for children, can stand without the sanction of science.

Children's Lunches

In the chapter on vitamin B we pointed out the value of peanut butter. It will bear reiteration. Milk and thick peanut-butter sandwiches of whole-wheat bread, supplemented by tomatoes or oranges, constitute an excellent lunch from the nutritional point of view. After peanut butter, meat and cheese, in that order, are the most nutritious sandwich fillers.

Recently the author analyzed a number of lunches which children brought to school in Pasadena. In the course of a week one child brought the following sixteen items: bread, butter, potato chips, chicken, bacon, mayonnaise, apple, banana, fruit salad, cooked peaches, strawberries, raisins, jelly, tomato, lettuce, and cake. Making a reasonable allowance for the amount of the day's food which might be in the lunch, this child's diet was deficient in calcium and phosphate. It was adequate, without being abundant, in vitamin A and thiamine (vitamin B_1).

Another child brought only six items in the course of the week: milk, bread, butter, mixed fruit salad, peanut butter, and carrots. This lunch was adequate in every respect.

The contribution of items such as celery, head lettuce, radishes, raisins, a few prunes, to the nutritional value of a lunch is trivial.

If butter is too expensive it can be replaced by margarine which contains added vitamin A. The margarines with added vitamin A on the market today contain about half the vitamin A of summer butter. If margarine is used, this difference in vitamin A can be made up by a few sprigs of parsley or a small extra helping of spinach or carrots.

The Diet for Adults

The best diet for adults is that recommended for children, with a few modifications. One pint of milk is sufficient. Most adults in the United States eat too much carbohydrate—starches and sweets. And they require more vitamin B than most of them get.

Adults have neither the time, the inclination, or, frequently, the facilities to take the little trouble necessary to obtain a good diet. To achieve anything in this direction the prescription must be as simple as possible.

For breakfast we recommend especially the use of the cereal, "the scalp of the sizings." Many of the nationally advertised breakfast foods provide very little for the money, apart from the taste. Almost their only value is as a vehicle for milk, cream, or fruit. Their vitamin content is low, and for calories they are very expensive. Oatmeal, especially if it contains the whole grain, is better than these advertised breakfast foods, but it is not so good as "the scalp of the sizings." Farina with added wheat germ is a good cereal. But it is usually difficult to obtain, and it may be more expensive than "the scalp of the sizings."

Five squares of butter provide too many calories for those who wish to keep their weight down. The chief value of butter in the diet of adults is its vitamin A. If butter is taboo for calorific reasons, the vitamin A can be obtained by eating more green leafy vegetables or by using vitamin A concentrates (capsules).

Margarines nowadays contain a significant amount of vitamin A and sometimes also vitamin D. These are almost as good as butter, and if they are cheaper they may be used without any qualms when the family budget is limited.

Some adults object to eating every morning the vitamin B rich cereal recommended. For variety, they can eat this cereal as biscuits, muffins, and pancakes. If that is not possible, then the only alternatives are one to one and one-half ounces of dried brewer's yeast daily or a liquid vitamin B concentrate. Some vitamin B supplement is essential. The ordinary good diet does not provide enough. Whether the supplement used is a cereal, yeast, or liquid concentrate, the amount taken should provide about 750 International Units of thiamine (vitamin B_1). There is, of course, no reason against using cereal and liquid concentrate at the same time, or cereal and yeast in order to reduce the amount of cereal to be eaten. For most families the liquid vitamin B concentrates are too expensive as the chief source of vitamin B.

It has been found that many cases of chronic gastrointestinal disorder are benefited when the following simple and practical rules are observed:

> *Eat no bread, either whole wheat or white.*
> *No potatoes, pie, or pastry.*
> *Drink daily one pint of milk, preferably "vitamin D" milk, pasteurized, as a drink or cooked (in soups, cocoa, chocolate, etc.).*
> *Eat daily at least one egg, not raw; best well cooked.*
> *Drink one tumblerful of some citrus juice or tomato juice daily.*

Drink four glasses of water daily.

Eat fresh meat once a day, with liberal servings of green vegetables; carrots and leafy vegetables such as broccoli or spinach at least once every day. For salads, instead of head lettuce use watercress, romaine lettuce, and parsley.

In cooking vegetables, use as little water as possible and do not throw it away; take it in some way with the food.

Try to obtain five squares of butter daily.

If you want more to eat, fill up on vegetables, meat, milk, and cheese.

In general, those desserts are better in which little sugar, starch, or pastry is used. Fruits, raw or cooked, are to be preferred, and better raw than cooked.

Do not take enemata or laxatives.

Supplement this diet with at least 750 International Units of vitamin B, daily from some *natural* source, e.g., "scalp of the sizings" or vitamin B-complex sirup.

Weight-Reducing Diets

When dietary weight reduction is attempted by a lay-woman, or under the direction of a faddist or charlatan, usually there is not only undernutrition but also serious malnutrition. This is what is wrong with the "Hollywood diet," fruit juice diets, and the like. The first and most important principle to be borne in mind here is that the quality of the diet must be maintained regardless of how drastically the quantity is reduced. Adequate amounts of the necessary vitamins and minerals, and some animal protein, must be provided.

The vitamins can be obtained as concentrates—one capsule containing enough of vitamins A and D, and two or three teaspoonfuls of a good liquid vitamin B complex concentrate. Pills, capsules, tablets, and concentrates advertised to contain vitamins A, B, D, and G, do not, as a rule, contain enough of the vitamin B complex. A glass of whole milk, an egg, and a half-glass of orange juice (four ounces) daily will supply minerals, fourteen grams of animal protein, and an adequate amount of vitamin C. All together these give only 330 calories. With this provision there is no danger of malnutrition. This is probably sufficient instruction for those who are not fat, but who wish to be or remain slim. Mirror, scales, and appetite will attend to the rest.

It will be unfortunate if the information above encourages anyone to undertake a drastic weight reduction by dieting without consulting a physician. This is not merely the author's medical trade unionism. There are many good reasons for this warning, too many to be enumerated in detail. Serious medical conditions must be excluded. The cause of the obesity, if it is obesity, must be determined if possible. There may be another, much more efficient and important remedy for the obesity than diet restriction. The amounts of the different foods to be eaten must be carefully prescribed. The drawing up of a drastic reducing regimen which will be efficient and safe requires expert knowledge of nutrition and medicine and a good deal of experience.

CHAPTER XI

Buying Vitamins

Vitamins for Sale

IN THE foregoing chapters it has frequently been suggested that the reader needs to exercise some care in finding the most economical source of one or another of the vitamins. The problem here is the old one of trying to get our money's worth. So far as the natural foods are concerned, seasonal and geographical variations in price, as well as personal preferences, make it almost impossible to lay down any principles for general guidance.

But when we want a vitamin supplement for the ordinary diet, it is possible to state a few simple rules which always should be followed.

No vitamin concentrate of any kind should be bought unless the potency is stated in terms of units in a given volume—cubic centimeter, gram, ounce, or drop.

With this information given and the aid of a little arithmetic, one product or another can be chosen very simply on the basis of price.[1] The products of reputable pharmaceutical houses state this information on the label.

---

[1] *If the prospective buyer encounters two different brands of the same vitamin concentrate, with the potency given in different systems of units, he will find that the conversion table on page 178 will enable him to convert them all, for purposes of comparison, into the same unit.*

*Concentrates containing vitamins A, B, C, and D in a single
preparation are not economical buys.*

Concentrates of vitamins A and D are cheap; those of
vitamins B and C are dear. In the usual mixtures there are
large amounts of the cheap A and D, and unimportant
amounts of the relatively expensive B and C.

Since the synthesized vitamins are by their nature standardized as to potency, the only factor to be taken into
account in buying them is advantageous price.

The New Gold Rush

With the increase of public interest in vitamins, it is only
to be expected that various large-scale business enterprises
should be alert to cash in on the general desire to benefit
from this latest scientific achievement. Already, numerous
commercial products are basing their advertising on "vitamin
appeal." We have commented on this in connection with
soaps and cosmetics.

Quite recently, soft drinks and packaged breakfast foods
have been bidding for customers on the basis of the vitamins
they contain. One typical advertisement shows a happy
family assembled at the breakfast table. They are happy
presumably because they know that their breakfast cereal
is enriched with vitamins A, B_1, D, and G, and, according
to the text, "with the additional vitamins present in 4 ounces
of orange juice and 10 ounces of milk" they will have "40
per cent of the day's minimum requirements of the five key
vitamins" A, B_1, C, D, and G.

But the 4 ounces of orange juice and the 10 ounces of milk

would give them practically the same amount of vitamins anyway; consequently, one wonders what the use is of bothering about the cereal. Another thing to note is that 40 per cent of the day's *minimum* requirements is all that is promised, while one of the fundamental points which the author has been trying to make all through this book is that the minimum requirement, while it will prevent deficiency disease, is still far below the amount necessary for abundant health. And, finally, the advertisement does not state either the minimum requirement or the vitamin content of the cereal.

Another advertisement is even worse. It assures the reader that the breakfast cereal in question gives him "the full vitamin B_1 content of choice white corn—nature's richest corn source of this precious element." Now it may very well be true that white corn is nature's richest corn source of vitamin B_1, but what the advertisement fails to add is that whole unprocessed corn—whether white or any other color— is only a fair source of vitamin B_1; it contains, for example, only about one-half of the B_1 of whole wheat.

There is no need of citing other examples; the popular magazines that the reader sees will supply plenty more. Such advertising steers clear of downright misrepresentation; it misrepresents only by inference.

This is not to say that the vitamin enrichment of commercial food products is in itself a bad thing. "Vitamin D" milk and margarine fortified with vitamins A or D have already been recommended. But with these the buyer knows exactly what he is getting in terms of vitamin content per quart or pound. Until he is given the same information about commercial food products nationally advertised for their vitamin qualities, he should be wary of them. If he likes them for other reasons, well and good, but their alleged vitamin potency had better be left out of account. And if he is asked to pay a higher price for such food products because of their undefined vitamin enrichment, he can be fairly certain that he is not getting his money's worth.

CHAPTER XII

Epilogue

OUR knowledge of vitamins now is sufficient to establish nutrition for the first time on a really scientific basis. We know how, by means of vitamins, to prevent serious deficiency diseases or, if they unhappily have got a start, how to cure them. More important for most of us, we know how, by means of vitamins, to regulate our daily diet so as to maintain a high level of general health as far as nutrition can do so—a state in which we feel the vigor and zest for life and work that come from a continued sense of physical well-being.

What vitamins can lead to beyond this is still somewhat in the realm of speculation. But already they have given us new insights into the chemistry of the human body. These have resulted from investigations of the part that vitamins play in physiological processes. As this research proceeds—and as similar lines of inquiry are followed in such fields as the ductless glands—it is altogether likely that we shall have to revise our fundamental ideas not only of human physiology but of human nature itself.

A final example, again from the author's own experience, may make this clearer. A man visibly in great pain called on me. He had heard of our work on vitamin B and he hoped that vitamin B might help him. He brought with him for me to read a newspaper article on the use of vitamin B_1 in neuritis. He knew the name of his disease, "tick dollaroo."

It is actually a French name, *tic douloureux*, but hardly anybody calls it that. This disease is the most painful form of facial neuralgia.

Tic douloureux has only one sign—pain. It is excruciating pain which starts at a sensitive point on the face, called the trigger point, and shoots or stabs like lightning through the face. The pain is sharply limited by the parts of the face and head innervated by the fifth cranial nerve. It is painful for these people to eat or talk. A breath of wind, the lightest touch, on the trigger point provokes a paroxysm of pain.

The disease is situated somewhere along the connections between the fifth cranial nerve and the higher brain centers. The damage is so slight that nothing is found on autopsy.

Probably the best palliative treatment of tic douloureux is alcohol injection of the nerve. The alcohol temporarily destroys the nerve and the pain stops until the nerve regenerates. Then the pain returns. Another palliative treatment is inhalation of a substance called trethylene. The radical treatment is a brain operation. The disease never cures itself.

I told my visitor that tic douloureux was a different neuritis from the kinds in which vitamin B_1 has been found useful. There was no reason to believe that vitamin B_1 would help him. On the other hand, I assured him it could not possibly do him any harm. If he was willing to try it, I would supply the material. Since nothing could be expected from the ordinary nutritional doses of vitamin B_1, I proposed giving him partly by mouth, mostly by intravenous injection, about ten times a good nutritional dose daily. He had to undertake on his part not to resort to any other form of treatment for relief of his pain, regardless of how bad it became. He agreed.

To my surprise, he reported two weeks after treatment

was begun that the pain was definitely less. It so happened that he had another illness at the same time which needed urgent treatment, and his physician wanted the vitamin B₁ treatment stopped. This was done. In a few weeks the pain was as severe as it had been before. This was very interesting, and I naturally wanted to know whether or not the temporary relief was a complete coincidence.

To answer this question a small clinic was established in the Kerckhoff Biological Laboratory at the California Institute of Technology. Dr. M. Y. Kremers and Dr. C. G. Wiggins joined the author in this study. Tic douloureux is said to be a rare disease. From the number of applications for treatment we have had it seems to be more common than is generally supposed. There may be several hundred thousand cases in the United States.

The reasons for undertaking this study at the Kerckhoff Biological Laboratory of the California Institute of Technology, which is not primarily concerned with medical research, exemplify the new and enlarged possibilities opened up for medicine and physiology by identification of the precise chemical nature of the vitamins and their subsequent artificial synthesis. This study would not have been undertaken if vitamin B₁ had not been available in pure form so that it could be administered in massive doses intravenously. It is impossible to eat every day enough of even the richest source of vitamin B₁ to obtain the massive doses we wished to give. Further, with pure synthetic vitamin, we can be sure that the results obtained can be attributed with certainty to the vitamin administered. When the vitamin is obtained from a food, it may be difficult to tell whether the effects observed are caused by the known vitamins or by other as yet unknown substances.

The idea we set out to test in our study of tic douloureux ran somewhat as follows: We now know that the different members of the vitamin B complex constitute parts of the chemical machinery of all nerve cells. Is it possible that by offering a damaged nerve cell a chance to enlarge its chemical apparatus, by presenting to it enormous doses of the vitamin B complex, this damaged cell will thereby be enabled to overcome a disease process, which it is unable to do with only normal amounts of chemical apparatus?

Further, sufferers from tic douloureux are excellent experimental material for the study of the physiology of pain—about which we possess very little scientific information. The disease is essentially the same in every case, thus meeting the first essential requirement of a suitable object for a physiological experiment. The disease is always restricted to the part of the face and head innervated by the fifth cranial nerve, and in about 96 per cent of cases is only on one side. The symptom—pain—is the same in every case. Pain is a subjective phenomenon; these sufferers are good objects for this study, because they can tell us the way they feel.

Since this study was begun in April 1938, some fifty-eight cases have been studied. In July 1940, thirty-seven were markedly improved—that is, completely free of pain or discomfort; fifteen were definitely improved; three were slightly improved; and only three derived no relief at all. It now seems that relief will be gained as long as the treatment is continued.

Biotechnology, in this instance application of our new knowledge regarding vitamins, not only provides us with the cure of widespread, serious nutritional disease, but promises to lead us to a deeper insight into the action of the nervous system, and to give us new therapeutic agents for diseases of the nervous system. It has already been mentioned that the site of the disease tic douloureux probably is the brain. Since massive doses of vitamin B are useful in the alleviation of this disease, it may be that other forms of nerve disease, for which there is no treatment at present, including some psychiatric disturbances, may respond also, because the action of vitamin B on nerve tissue is general and not specific to any one group of nerve cells.

More than this: we know the precise chemical reactions which are controlled by the vitamins of the B complex. If tic douloureux responds to massive doses of vitamin B_1, then we may be able to make an important step forward in neurology, to restate the scientific description of a disease of the nervous system in terms of definite, precise chemical reactions. We shall have learned something of the chemical basis of one of our sensations.

But even more than this, advances in biology and biotechnology help to free us from prejudice and superstition, for they contribute toward a rational interpretation of life and of man's place in the world.

It was a wonderfully stimulating and encouraging discovery that the vitamins, substances which in minute amounts constitute indispensable parts of the chemical apparatus of all living cells, are really rather simple chemicals. This discovery places a profound understanding of the chemical basis of life well within our grasp. There can be no doubt that a large part of the physiology and pathology of the nervous system will be restated in terms of chemical reactions. Important members of the chemical machinery of the nervous system have already been worked out. The cure of beri-beri or polyneuritis by vitamin B_1, and the return of sanity to pellagrins after treatment with nicotinic acid and the B complex, point the way in which we can go and are going.

Sooner or later the experimental embryologist will discover the forces that determine the direction in which nerves grow in the development of the brain. We shall then understand how it comes about that we think as we do, how certain behavior patterns are inherited. It is not improbable that the embryologist will discover chemical and physical methods for at least modifying this nerve pattern in the central nervous system. We shall then have some insight into the chemical and physical and mechanical reasons for our being what we are, and for what happens when we or others do not behave as we wish.

Our understanding and judgment of personal behavior will then be on a more rational, more objectively defined basis than it is now. Tolerance will be less of a strain, because with an understanding of the physiological reason for an action we disapprove of we can more easily do something effective about it, not only to the other fellow, but to ourselves.

This change will certainly profoundly influence our notions of misbehavior. Lest this seem unwarrantably iconoclastic, we may recall that some instances of aberrant behavior are now considered, even in the courts, not as cases of moral obliquity or crime deserving punishment, but as manifestations of disease requiring treatment. As time goes on, we shall think less and less in terms of misbehavior and more and more in terms of physiology and chemistry.

As time goes on, in a better sense than Sganarelle's, we shall be changing all that.

SUMMARY DIGEST

Chief Common Sources of the Vitamins

The text should be consulted for explanatory details and the tables on pages 179 to 192 for the numerical data. It will be convenient to use this digest as a guide to the tables.

VITAMIN A

Fish-liver oils
Liver
Egg-yolk
Butter
Whole milk

Green leafy
      vegetables
Brussels sprouts
Green peas
Sweet potatoes
Apricots

Papayas
Prunes
Yellow peaches
Yellow cornmeal
Green stringbeans

VITAMIN B₁ (THIAMINE)

Whole grain cereals
Whole wheat bread
Wheat germ
"Scalp of the
      sizings"
  (see page 70)
Milk
Chicken
Ham

Lean pork
Brussels sprouts
Bananas (for
      children)
Cantaloupe
Grapefruit
Tomatoes
Dried beans (lima,
  navy, soy)

Green lima beans
Endive
Peas
Potatoes
Peanuts
Peanut butter
Yeast
Liver

VITAMIN C

Beet tops
Broccoli
Brussels sprouts

Cabbage (raw)
Cauliflower
Kale

Kohlrabi
Parsnips
Potatoes

Spinach
Watercress
Avocado
Bananas (for
    children)
Currants

Grapefruit
Lemons
Oranges
Papayas
Peppers

Raspberries
Strawberries
Tangerines
Tomatoes
Tomato juice

Vitamin B₂

Liver
Kidney
Lean meat
Crab
Fish
Oysters
Eggs
Cottage cheese

Milk
Beets
Carrots
Green leafy
        vegetables
Dried beans
Peas
Avocado

Peaches
Pears
Prunes
Tomatoes
Peanuts
Yeast
Wheat germ

Vitamin D

There are no good sources of vitamin D in common foods; hence the necessity of using commercial fish-liver oils. Small, but unimportant amounts are present in egg-yolk, salmon, sardines, milk, and butter.

Vitamin E

Egg-yolk
Muscle and body fat
Spinach
Watercress

Green leafy vege-
    tables especially
    lettuce (green)
Embryo of cereals

Vegetable oils
    (cottonseed,
    corn, palm)

"Vitamin F"

Corn oil
Linseed oil
Olive oil

Poppy-seed oil
Tung oil
Egg-yolk

Very widely dis-
    tributed in foods.

Vitamin K

Green leaves   Green cabbage   Spinach

Probably synthesized by bacteria in the human intestine.

Daily Human Vitamin Requirements for Abundant Health

VITAMIN A: *child:* 3000 International units

            adult: 6000 International units

VITAMIN B_1 (Thiamine Chloride):

        child: 10 International units per pound of body weight

        adult: 5–7 International units per pound of body weight

VITAMIN C: *baby:* 10 milligrams

        child: 3–4 milligrams per pound of body weight

        adult: 1 milligram per pound of body weight; 40 milligrams daily will prevent scurvy

VITAMIN D: *child until adolescence:* 1000 International (or U.S.P.) units

        adult: requirement not known as yet

VITAMIN B_2: *child:* 1.3–1.8 milligrams

        adult: 2.0–2.5 milligrams

III

Examples of a Day's Food for Children and Adults at Different Price Levels

The following tables are examples of a day's food for children and adults. They show that an abundance of vitamins may be obtained on a restricted food budget as well as when the cost of food is unimportant.

Substitutions can be made, with the tables on pages 179 to **193** as a guide, according to taste, availability at the time, and cost.

These food lists give only the important sources of vitamins. It is understood that the following will be eaten also: sugar, confections, cake, relishes, and beverages, as well as those fruits and vegetables which may be unimportant as sources of vitamins but are enjoyable.

In some instances it may be more convenient or more desirable to substitute vitamin concentrates or synthetic vitamins in the form of pills. According to the amounts taken in this form, the vitamins in the food may be more or less ignored. The table of the quantities of the different vitamins required, page 165, will be a guide.

There are other indispensable dietary factors besides vitamins—calories, protein, some fat, and minerals. Pills and concentrates cannot supply them all. They must be obtained from the natural foods.

For those vegetables which are usually eaten cooked, the vitamin values given are for cooked vegetables with all the water retained.

A Sample

Where the Fo

Items not important as sources of vita

BOY (7 OR 8
GIRL (8 TO

Item	Quantity
APPLE PIE	1/2 section
BANANA, baked	1
BEANS, dried lima	1/4 cup
BEEF, stewed steak	1/4 pound
BEET TOPS (chard)	1/4 cup
BREAD, 100% whole wheat	4 slices
EGG	1
LETTUCE, green	1 large leaf
MARGARINE (with added Vitamin A)	4 squares
MILK, whole	1 quart
OATMEAL	1/2 cup (dry)
PEANUT BUTTER	2 tablespoonfuls
POTATO	1/2 medium-sized
TOMATOES, canned	1/4 cup
Totals	

Alternatives

Item	Quantity
BEET ROOTS, cooked or canned	1/2 cup
CABBAGE (raw) used as cole slaw	1 cup
CARROTS	1/2 cup
CORN, yellow, canned	1/2 cup
POTATOES, sweet	1 medium-sized
SPINACH	1/2 cup
SQUASH, Hubbard	1/2 cup

Where

Items not im

Item
BEEF, top round
BREAD, 100% whole wheat
BUTTER
EGG
LETTUCE, romaine
MAYONNAISE
MILK, whole
PEAS, fresh
POTATO, baked
OATMEAL
ORANGE JUICE
STRAWBERRIES
TOMATOES
WATERCRESS
Totals

CHEESE, American
CARROTS
PEANUT BUTTER
"SCALP OF SIZINGS" (see page 70)
SPINACH

A Sample of a Day's Food, the Cost of Food Does Not Matter

ortant as sources of vitamins—sugar, confections, relishes, beverages—are omitted.

	BOY (7 OR 8 YEARS) OR GIRL (8 TO 10 YEARS)				MODERATELY ACTIVE MAN		
Quantity	Vitamin A	Vitamin B₁	Vitamin C	Quantity	Vitamin A	Vitamin B₁	Vitamin C
	International Units	International Units	Milligrams		International Units	International Units	Milligrams
1/4 pound	40	45	2	3/4 pound	120	135	6.5
4 slices	280	108	0	4 slices	280	108	0
4 squares	1,260	0	0	5 squares	1,575	0	0
1	900	19	0	1	900	19	0
1 long leaf	650	2	0.5	2 long leaves	1,300	4	1
2 tablespoonfuls	60	1	0	2 tablespoonfuls	60	1	0
1 quart	1,400	150	19	1 pint	700	75	9.5
1/3 cup	350	52	9	1/2 cup	530	78	13
1/2 medium-sized	20	30	8	1 medium-sized	40	60	15
1/2 cup (dry)	0	130	0	1/2 cup (dry)	0	130	0
1 glass (6 ounces)	540	59	98	1 glass (6 ounces)	540	59	98
1/3 box	230	0	63	1/2 box	340	0	93
1/2 medium-sized	2,650	13	13	1/2 medium-sized	2,650	13	13
1/3 bunch	1,350	19	15	1/2 bunch	2,000	28	22
	9,730	628	227.5		11,035	710	271

Alternatives

2 one-inch cubes	840	6	0
1/2 cup	1,350	16	2.5
2 tablespoonfuls	17	125	0
1/2 cup (dry)	200	260	0
1/2 cup	14,000	30	26

Vitamin Content of
a Day's Food
of a Four-Year-Old Child

(day I on page 173)

Item	Quantity	Vitamin A	Vitamin B_1	Vitamin C
		International Units	International Units	Milligrams
APPLE BETTY	2 tablespoonfuls	22	4	0
APRICOTS, canned	2 halves	1,000	2	1
BEET TOPS, cooked	1/2 tablespoonful	1,200	2	4
BREAD, 100% whole wheat	3 slices	210	81	0
BUTTER	3 squares	945		
CEREAL, "scalp of sizings"	1/4 cup (dry)	100	130	0
GRAHAM CRACKERS	2	26	8	0
LAMB CHOP	2 French chops or 1 shoulder chop	0	45	1
MILK	1 quart	1,400	150	19
ORANGE JUICE	1/2 cup	360	40	48
PARSLEY	4 stems	1,000		11
PEANUT BUTTER	1 tablespoonful	8	65	0
POTATO, mashed	1/2 potato	20	29	7
RICE, brown, creamed	1/4 cup	62	19	1
Totals		6,353	575	92

Vitamins for Those

AN AVERAGE DAY'S RESTAURANT MENU

Item	Quantity	Vita-min A	Vita-min B₁	Vita-min C
		Inter-national Units	Inter-national Units	Milli-grams
Breakfast				
TOMATO JUICE	small glass	2,650	12	12
HOT CAKES	2	400	22	0
SIRUP	small pitcher	0	0	0
BUTTER	2 squares	630	0	0
COFFEE		0	0	0
Lunch				
TUNA-FISH SANDWICH on white bread				
⎰tuna fish		0	8	0
⎱bread		20	7	0
BUTTER	1 square	315	0	0
CHOCOLATE MILK SHAKE	large glass (12 ounces)	0	37	4
Dinner				
VEGETABLE SOUP	1 cup	113	9	4
STEAK	1 serving	40	45	2
POTATOES, mashed	1 serving	60	58	15
STRINGBEANS	1 serving	600	17	4
BREAD, white	2 slices	20	7	0
BUTTER	1 square	315	0	0
COFFEE		0	0	0
Totals		5,163	222	41

Who Eat in Restaurants

EASY SUBSTITUTIONS
Which Will Provide
a Richer Vitamin Intake at
Little or No Increase in Cost

Item	Quantity	Vita- min A	Vita- min B₁	Vita- min C
		Inter- national Units	Inter- national Units	Milli- grams

Breakfast

Item	Quantity	Vitamin A	Vitamin B₁	Vitamin C
ORANGE JUICE	small glass	270	30	36
BREAD, 100% whole wheat	1 slice	75	27	0
BUTTER	1 square	315	0	0
BACON	2 strips	0	2	0
EGG	1	900	19	0

Lunch

Item	Quantity	Vitamin A	Vitamin B₁	Vitamin C
HAM SANDWICH ON 100% whole wheat bread				
ham		0	120	0
bread		140	54	0
BUTTER	1 square	315	0	0
MILK	1 glass (6 ounces)	260	28	3.5

Dinner

Item	Quantity	Vitamin A	Vitamin B₁	Vitamin C
SALAD lettuce	2 leaves	500	8	2
tomato	1/2	3,000	26	25
STEAK	1 serving	40	45	2
POTATOES, mashed	1 serving	60	58	15
STRINGBEANS	1 serving	600	17	4
BREAD, 100% whole wheat	1 slice	70	27	0
BUTTER	1 square	315	0	0
MILK	1 glass (6 ounces)	260	28	35
		7,120	489	122.5

Alternatives

When fresh tomatoes are out of season, canned tomato juice is a good substitute. Other, somewhat inferior, alternatives are cole slaw (raw cabbage) and sliced beets.

Menus for Children

Below is the list of twenty-one meals for a child, which I
flinched from imposing on my daughter. But the publishers, who
are made of sterner stuff, requested these menus.

The quantities given are for a four-year-old child; they will, of
course, be adjusted up and down for older and younger children.
Older children will require more meat and fish. Adolescent children need as much as or even more food than adults.

This dietary provides adequate amounts of vitamins (except
vitamin D) and of minerals, calories, protein, carbohydrate, and
fat. The milk is preferably "Vitamin D" milk.

These menus should be adapted so that they will be made up
of foods which the whole family is eating. The noon and evening
meals may be interchanged if too heavy a meal does not interfere
with the child's sleep.

A fish-liver oil rich in vitamin D should be provided especially
during the winter months and even in the summer if the child has
little chance to be in the sunshine.

Milk may be used as such and in milk and vegetable soups,
cocoa, milk toast, milk sherbets, junkets, custards.

It should not be forgotten that milk is filling. If the child com-
plains that he is unable to eat all his food, the milk may be given
toward the end of the meal or the amount reduced temporarily;
or powdered milk or evaporated milk may be used in cooking to
provide the milk solids without increasing the bulk of the diet too
much.

Menus for a Four-Year-Old Child

<table>
<tr><td colspan="2">

I

MORNING MEAL

</td><td colspan="2">

II

MORNING MEAL

</td></tr>
<tr>
<td>Orange juice</td><td>1/2 cup</td>
<td>Banana, baked</td><td></td>
</tr>
<tr>
<td>"Scalp of sizings"</td><td>1/4 cup (dry)</td>
<td>Oatmeal and "scalp</td><td></td>
</tr>
<tr>
<td>100% whole wheat</td><td></td>
<td>of sizings" mixed</td><td></td>
</tr>
<tr>
<td>bread</td><td>1 slice</td>
<td>in equal parts</td><td>1/4 cup (dry)</td>
</tr>
<tr>
<td>Butter</td><td>1 pat or square</td>
<td>100% whole wheat</td><td></td>
</tr>
<tr>
<td>Milk</td><td>1 quart per day</td>
<td>bread</td><td>1 slice</td>
</tr>
<tr>
<td></td><td></td>
<td>Butter</td><td>1 pat or square</td>
</tr>
<tr>
<td></td><td></td>
<td>Milk</td><td>1 quart per day</td>
</tr>
</table>

NOON MEAL

I		II	
Lamb chops	2 French chops or 1 shoulder chop	Stringbeans	1 1/2 table-spoonfuls
Beet tops	1/2 tablespoon-ful cooked	Baked sweet potato	1 small
		Cottage cheese on	1 heaping
Mashed potato	1/2 potato	lettuce leaf	tablespoonful
Parsley and peanut		Pineapple	1/2 large ring
butter sandwich		Custard	1/2 custard cup
Apple Betty	2 tablespoons	100% whole wheat	
Milk		bread	1 slice
		Butter	1 pat or square
		Milk	

4:00 p.m.

Milk and 2 graham crackers

4:00 p.m.

Orange juice (1/2 glass) and
2 graham crackers

EVENING MEAL

I		II	
		Creamed vegetable	
		soup	1/2 cup
		Crackers	2
Creamed brown rice	1/4 cup	Stewed dried	
100% whole wheat		peaches	1/4 cup
bread	1 slice	100% whole wheat	
Butter	1 pat or square	bread	1 slice
Apricots	2	Butter	1 pat or square
Milk		Milk	

III

Morning Meal

Orange juice	1/2 glass
"Scalp of sizings"	1/4 cup (dry)
100% whole wheat bread	1 slice
Butter	1 pat or square
Milk	1 quart per day

Noon Meal

Creamed eggs	2
Spinach	1 1/2 table-spoonfuls
Carrot strips	1 tablespoonful
Brown rice pudding	1/2 cup
100% whole wheat bread	1 slice
Butter	1 pat or square
Milk	

4:00 p.m.

Milk and 2 graham crackers

Evening Meal

Yellow cornmeal mush	1/4 cup dry, 1 cup cooked
Stewed fruit com-pote	1/2 cup
100% whole wheat bread	1 slice
Butter	1 pat or square
Milk	

IV

Morning Meal

Orange juice	1/2 cup
"Scalp of sizings"	1/4 cup (dry)
100% whole wheat bread	1 slice
Butter	1 pat or square
Milk	1 quart per day

Noon Meal

Liver	1 small serving
Creamed potatoes or 1/2 potato	1/4 cup
Asparagus	5 stalks
Zwieback	3 pieces
Butter	1 pat or square
Cookies	2 or 3
Milk	

4:00 p.m.

Milk and 2 graham crackers

Evening Meal

Creamed tomato soup	1/2 cup
100% whole wheat bread	1 slice
Butter	1 pat or square
Stewed fruit	1/2 cup
Milk	

V

MORNING MEAL

Baked apple	1/2
Oatmeal and "scalp of sizings" mixed in equal parts	1/4 cup (dry)
100% whole wheat bread	1 slice
Butter	1 pat or square
Milk	1 quart per day

NOON MEAL

Scrambled egg	1
Tomato	1/2
Carrots, buttered	1 1/2 table-spoonfuls
Lettuce and parsley sandwich with 100% whole wheat bread and butter	1
Grapenut pudding	1/4 cup

4:00 p.m.

Milk and 2 graham crackers

EVENING MEAL

Creamed celery soup	1/2 cup
Zwieback	3 pieces
Butter	1 pat or square
Pear	1/2
Milk	

VI

MORNING MEAL

Prune purée	1/4 cup
"Scalp of sizings"	1/4 cup (dry)
Coddled egg	1
100% whole wheat bread	1 slice
Butter	1 pat or square
Milk	1 quart per day

NOON MEAL

Creamed spinach	1/4 cup
Baked potato	1 small
Celery stalk	2 branches
100% whole wheat bread	1 slice
Butter	1 pat or square
Spanish cream	
Milk	

4:00 p.m.

Orange juice (1/2 glass) and 2 graham crackers

EVENING MEAL

Wheatena	2/3 cup cooked
Zwieback	3 pieces
Butter	1 pat or square
Stewed peaches	1/4 cup
Milk	

VII

Morning Meal		Noon Meal	
Pear	1/2	Liver loaf	1 medium serving
Oatmeal and "scalp of sizings" mixed in equal parts	1/4 cup (dry)	Creamed potato with parsley	1/2 potato
100% whole wheat bread	1 slice	Buttered peas	1/4 cup
		100% whole wheat	
Butter	1 pat or square	bread	1 slice
Milk	1 quart per day	Butter	1 pat or square
		Ice cream	1 helping
		Milk	

4:00 p.m.

Orange juice (1/2 glass) and
2 graham crackers

Evening Meal

Milk toast (whole wheat)	3 slices
Peanut butter and lettuce sandwich with buttered 100% whole wheat bread	1
Stewed prunes	1/4 cup

This list of menus was prepared by Miss C. Knudson under the direction of Miss L. Giebelstein, dietitian of the Food Clinic, Los Angeles County General Hospital. The selection of foods is based on the vitamin contents of foods on pages 179 to 193 and additional data on the mineral contents of foods compiled by the author.

V

The Vitamin Contents of Common Foods

Unless otherwise indicated, the quantities given below are those in the dry or fresh state before cooking.[1]

No values for vitamin D are given because except in milk, butter, and eggs, the amounts in all foods are negligible. Even in these three foods the amounts are so small that commercially prepared concentrates of vitamin D must be used.

The data are as yet too scanty, or the daily human requirement is inadequately determined, to make it useful to include in this table values of vitamins B_6, nicotinic acid, pantothenic acid, E, and K.

The figures in parentheses are estimates based on figures obtained from similar foods which have undergone similar treatment.

Where no vitamin values are given in the table it is because they have not yet been determined. In any case, the amount present probably is insignificant for ordinary nutritional purposes, except in the case of vitamin B_2.

---

[1] *There is little information on the effect of freezing operations on the vitamin content of foods except in the case of vitamin C. This vitamin is so easily destroyed that, for the time being, until more information is available, we may conservatively apply the findings in the case of vitamin C to all the other vitamins. Freezing itself, if it is done quickly, has no destructive action. Losses occur in the course of slow freezing, storage at temperatures above $0°F.$, and slow thawing. Cooking of frozen foods should be begun while they are still in the frozen condition. Fruits which are to be eaten uncooked should be served immediately after thawing.*

UNIT EQUIVALENTS

VITAMIN A

1 International unit = 2 Sherman units
= 0.6 microgram (gamma, γ) of β carotene

VITAMIN B₁ (THIAMINE CHLORIDE)

1 International unit = 3 micrograms (gamma, γ)
= 0.003 milligram
= 2 Sherman units

VITAMIN C (ASCORBIC ACID, CEVITAMIC ACID)

1 milligram = 20 International units
= 2 Sherman units

VITAMIN B₂ (RIBOFLAVIN)

1 milligram = 333 Sherman-Bourquin units
= 1000 micrograms (gamma, γ)

ABBREVIATIONS

I.U. = International units
Mg. = milligrams
tblsp. = tablespoonful
1 tumbler = common drinking glass containing 6 ounces

The symbol ″ after a number = inches. For example 1½″ = one and one-half inches.

MEASURE			Vitamin A	Vitamin B_1	Vitamin C	Vitamin B_2
Ordinary	Ounces		I. U. per Measure	I. U. per Measure	Milligrams per Measure	Milligrams per Measure

BREADS AND CEREALS

Barley, whole grain	1 tblsp.	1/2	0	3.3		0.001
" , pearled	1 tblsp.	1/2	0	0		
*Biscuits, baking powder	1 biscuit		19	3	0	
Bread, "Boston brown"	1 slice 3″ diam., 3/8″ thick	3/4	55	13	0	
" , white, made with milk	1 slice 3″ x 3 1/2″ x 1/2″	3/4	10	3.8	0	0.0121
" , white, made with water	1 slice 3″ x 3 1/2″ x 1/2″	3/4	10	3.7	0	0.006
" , 100% wheat	1 slice 3″ x 3″ x 3/8″	1	70	27	0	
" , rye	1 slice 3″ x 3″ x 3/8″	1		14		
Corn, whole grain, yellow	1 cup	5	1200	72	11	0.05
" , flakes (packaged cereal)	1 cup	1 1/3		trace	0	
" , meal, white	1 cup	5	0	143		
✓ " , meal, yellow	1 cup	5	1200	110		0.142
*Crackers, Graham	1 cracker		26	8	0	
✓ *Custard, baked	3/4 cup	3	650	21	1	
Flour, rye	1 cup	5		30–70		
" , 100% whole, unbleached	1 cup	4	500	180	0	
" , white, bleached	1 cup	4	150	33	0	
" , white, pastry or patent	1 cup	4	130	19	0	
" , white, plus germ	1 cup	4		49	0	
*Griddlecakes	1 medium	2	200	11	0.5	
*Muffins, plain, made with egg	1 muffin		135	9	0	
* " , plain, made without egg	1 muffin		48	8	0	
* " , bran, made with egg	1 muffin		260	52	0	
* " , bran, made without egg	1 muffin		170	50	0	

* These values have been calculated from typical home-cooking recipes. Commercial recipes will not contain more than the values given; for example, where recipes call for butter, it is possible that commercial preparations will use margarine, containing no vitamin A, or lard, and so on. The significance of this type of substitution is seen in the case of vegetable soup; more than half of the vitamin A indicated in the table comes from butter used in making the soup.

MEASURE Ordinary	Ounces	Vitamin A I.U. per Measure	Vitamin B₁ I.U. per Measure	Vitamin C Milligrams per Measure	Vitamin B₂ Milligrams per Measure

BREADS AND CEREALS *(Continued)*

Oatmeal, whole grain	1/2 cup	3/4	0	165	
" , prepared breakfast meal (quick-cooking)	1/2 cup	3/4	0	130	0
Oats, rolled, packaged	1/2 cup	3/4	0	121	0
" , rolled, cooked (double boiler)	1/2 cup	3/4	0	121	0
Rice, brown	2 tblsp.	1	17	15	0.02
" , polished	2 tblsp.	1	0	0	0.022
" , unpolished, boiled (dry weight)	2 tblsp.	1	0	0	0.035
" , ground	2 tblsp.	1		7	
*Rolls	1 roll	1 1/2	74	9	0
Rye, whole grain	1 cup	5		210	0
Wheat, whole grain	1 tblsp.	1/2	50	23	4	0.02
" , whole grain, cooked (double boiler)	1 tblsp.	1/2	50	23	
" , bran	1 tblsp.	1/2	85	28	0
" , farina, light	1 tblsp.	1/3	0	0.2	0	0
" , farina, dark	1 tblsp.	1/3	trace	7	0	0.02
" , germ	1 tblsp.	1/2	90	80	0	0.10
" , middlings, plus 15% germ ("scalp of the sizings." See page 70)	1 tblsp.	1/2	50	65		0.02
" , puffed	1/2 cup	1/2		0	0
" , semolina	1 tblsp.	1/2	30	7	
" , shredded	1 biscuit	1	4	20	0	0.10
Wheat, stone-ground	1 tblsp.	1/2	40	22	3	0.015

DAIRY PRODUCTS

Butter	1 square 1 1/4" x 1 1/4" x 1/4"	1/3	315	0	trace	0.001
Buttermilk	1 large glass	8	0	35	2	0.310
Cheese, American Cheddar	1" cube	3/4	420	3	0	0.12
" , Camembert	1" cube	3/4	750		0	

* These values have been calculated from typical home-cooking recipes.

MEASURE			Vitamin A	Vitamin B_1	Vitamin C	Vitamin B_2
Ordinary		Ounces	I.U. per Measure	I.U. per Measure	Milligrams per Measure	Milligrams per Measure

DAIRY PRODUCTS *(Continued)*

Food	Ordinary	Ounces	A	B_1	C	B_2
Cheese, cottage, skim milk	1 tblsp.	3/5	70		0	0.068
" , creamed, soft	1 tblsp.	1/2	310	0.6	0	0.017
" , creamed, full	piece 2″ x 1″ x 3/8″	1	500		0	0.02
" , Edam	1″ cube	3/4	300		0	
" , pimento (Kraft)	1″ cube	3/4	500			
" , Roquefort	1″ cube	3/4	850		0	
" , Swiss (Kraft)	slice 4″ x 4″ x 1/8″	3/4	440		0	
Cream, 20% fat	1 tblsp.	3/5	64	2	trace	
" , 40% fat	1 tblsp.	3/5	132	1.6	trace	
Eggs, whole	1 egg	1 1/2	900	19	0	0.25
" , white	1 white	9/10	0	trace	0	0.14
" , yolk	1 yolk	6/10	900	19	0	0.11
" , soft-boiled	1 egg	6/10	900	19	0	
" , hard-boiled	1 egg	6/10	900	19	0	
Milk, whole, fresh, raw	1 quart	32	1400	150	19	1.20
	1 glass	6	260	28	3.5	0.23
" , whole, fresh, pasteurized	1 glass	6	260	22	3.0	0.23
" , dried powder	1 tblsp.	1/4	70	7.3	0.7	0.07
" , dried, reconstituted	1 tumbler	6	260	20	2.0	0.20
" , evaporated	1/2 cup	4	190	15	3.5	0.35
" , condensed, sweetened	1 tblsp.	3/4	45	10		
" , skim, fresh	1 glass	6	trace	25	4.0	0.17
" , skim, dried powder	1 tblsp.	1/4	0	8	0.7	0.09
* " , shake, commercial ice cream and skim milk		12	0	37	4	

MEAT AND FISH

Food	Ordinary	Ounces	A	B_1	C	B_2
Bacon, fried	5 slices	1/2		5	0	
Beef, lean, top round	1/4 lb.	4	40	45	2.2	0.06
Beef, lean, stewed steak	1/4 lb.	4	20	18	1	
Chicken, light meat	1/4 lb.	4		30	0	0.029
" , dark meat	1/4 lb.	4		42	0	0.078

* These values have been calculated from typical home-cooking recipes.

MEASURE		Vitamin A	Vitamin B₁	Vitamin C	Vitamin B₂
Ordinary	Ounces	I. U. per Measure	I. U. per Measure	Milligrams per Measure	Milligrams per Measure

MEAT AND FISH (Continued)

	MEASURE Ordinary	Ounces	Vitamin A	Vitamin B₁	Vitamin C	Vitamin B₂
Chicken, dark meat, roasted	1/4 lb.	4		35	0	
" , liver*	1/8 lb.	2	17,000	50	11	2.0
Cod, steak, fresh	1/4 lb.	4	2	34	0	0.11
Crab	1/4 lb.	4	2200	45	5	0.40
Halibut, muscle, fresh	1/4 lb.	4		32		0.21
" , muscle, fried	1/4 lb.	4		30		
Ham, smoked, lean, raw	1/4 lb.	4		540		
" , smoked, lean, boiled	1/4 lb.	4		450		
Herring, whole	1/4 lb.	4	1700	20		0.12
" , whole, fried	1/4 lb.	4	(1500)	0		
Kidney, beef or calf	1/4 lb.	4	450	105	12	1.6
" , beef or calf, cooked (fried 10 minutes)	1/4 lb.	4	450	85	6	
Lamb, chop, lean	1/4 lb.	4	trace	90	2	
" , roasted	1/4 lb.	4	trace	60	1	
Liver,* beef, fresh	1/4 lb.	4	46,000	100	34	3.4
" , beef, fried, or boiled and water kept	1/4 lb.	4	46,000	100	28	
" , beef, boiled and water discarded	1/4 lb.	4	46,000	(50)	6	
Mackerel	1/4 lb.	4		34		
Mutton, lean	1/4 lb.	4		68		
Oysters, raw	1/3 cup	3 1/2	420	75	3	0.46
" , cooked	1/3 cup	3 1/2	300	60		
Pork, chop, lean	1/4 lb.	4	0	515	2	
" , chop, lean, braised	1/4 lb.	4	0	440	1	
" , loin, lean	1/4 lb.	4	0	515	2	0.28
" , loin, lean, roasted	1/4 lb.	4	0	290	1	
Prawns, boiled	1/4 lb.	4	1100	20	0	0.11
Rabbit, stewed	1/4 lb.	4		23	trace	0.07
Salmon, fresh, raw	1/4 lb.	4	200–500			
" , canned, red	1/4 lb.	4	340	trace		0.27
" , canned, pink	1/4 lb.	4	110	trace		0.27
" , Chinook	1/4 lb.	4	600	trace		0.27
" , Calico, chum	1/4 lb.	4	32	trace		0.27

* Vitamins eaten in chicken liver or in beef liver are retained fully, i.e., absorbed and assimilated and thereby made available to the body.

MEASURE		Vitamin A	Vitamin B₁	Vitamin C	Vitamin B₂
Ordinary	Ounces	I. U. per Measure	I. U. per Measure	Milligrams per Measure	Milligrams per Measure

MEAT AND FISH *(Continued)*

Sardines, canned in oil	1/8 lb.	2	200	17	
Sweetbreads, fresh	1/4 lb.	4		120	
" , fried	1/4 lb.	4		34	
Tongue, beef or sheep, cooked	1/4 lb.	4		35	
Tripe, stewed	1/4 lb.	4		15	
Trout, fresh-water	1/4 lb.	4		33	
Veal, muscle, cooked	1/4 lb.	4	40	45	2	0.17
Whiting, Atlantic, flesh	1/4 lb.	4	400		

FRUITS

Apples, raw, average common varieties	1 medium size	6	50	8	10	0.06
" , baked	1 medium size	6			3	
" , applesauce	1/2 cup	4 1/2			9	
" , juice	1 tumbler	6			5	
Apricots, fresh	1 medium	1 1/3	1000	3.5	2	0.04
" , canned	2 medium halves	1 1/4	1000	2	1	0.04
" , dried	4 halves	3/5	540	8	0	0.009
" , dried, sulphured	4 halves	3/5	540	3	2	0.005
Avocado, California	1/2 avocado	4	64	40	25	0.19
Bananas	1 medium	5 1/2	230	28	7	0.07
Blackberries	1 cup	5 3/4	230	10	15	
Blueberries	1 cup	5 1/4	150	21	8	0.021
Cantaloupe	1/2 melon 5" diam.	13 1/2	770	73	60	0.25
Cherries, fresh, Bing	10 cherries 7/8" diam.	2 1/3	75	12	13	
" , fresh, Royal Anne	10 cherries 7/8" diam.	2 1/3	130	(12)	13	
" , canned, Royal Anne	10 cherries	2 1/3	(100)	(10)	(10)	
Cranberries, fresh	1 cup	3 3/4	20	0	20	0
" , juice	1/2 cup	2			7	0
Currants, black, fresh	1 cup	3 3/4		11	220	
" , black, canned, not strained	1 cup	3 3/4		(8)	200	

MEASURE		Vitamin A	Vitamin B₁	Vitamin C	Vitamin B₂
Ordinary	Ounces	I. U. per Measure	I. U. per Measure	Milligrams per Measure	Milligrams per Measure

FRUITS *(Continued)*

Currants, black, canned, strained	1 cup	3 3/4		(6)	150
" , red, fresh	1 cup	3 3/4		16	55
" , red, canned, not strained	1 cup	3 3/4		(12)	40
" , red, canned, strained	1 cup	3 3/4		(10)	30
Dates, fresh	4 dates	1 1/2	35	12	0	0.012
" , dried, unstoned	4 dates	1 1/5	15	8.5	0	0
Figs, fresh	3 small	4	90	30	2.3	0.06
" , dried	3 small	2 1/5	32	30	0
Gooseberries, fresh	1 cup	4	330	56	34
" , canned, not strained	1 cup	4	330	(45)	34
" , canned and strained	1 cup	4	330	(25)	17
Grapefruit	1/2 medium	7 1/2	0	51	100
" , juice, fresh	1 tumbler	6	0	35	75	0.006
" , juice, canned	1 tumbler	6	0	35	75
Grapes (25–30)	1/2 bunch	4	22	11	2.2	0
" , Thompson seedless (25–30)	1/2 bunch	4	56	17	3.3	0
" , juice	1 tumbler	6	0	0	0	0
Guava (stoned)	1 guava	3/4	22	2	30	0.006
Lemon	1 large	3 3/5	0		55
" , juice	2 tblsp.	1	0		15	0.001
Lime, pulp	1 medium	2	100		20
" , juice, fresh	2 tblsp.	1	8		10
Mangoes	1 mango	3	850	17	25	0.05
Olives, green	6 olives	2	85	trace	0
" , ripe Manzanilla	6 olives	2	85	trace	0
" , ripe Mission	6 olives	2	28	trace	0
Orange, pulp	1 large	9 1/2	80–270	95	80	0.24
" , juice, fresh	1 tumbler	6	540	59	98	0.012
" , juice, canned	1 tumbler	6	(540)	(59)	72
Papayas	1 papaya	3	1800	7	46	0.015
Peaches, Elberta, fresh	1 medium	4	900	28	3.4	0.008
" , Elberta, canned	2 halves	3	(900)	22	(1.7)

MEASURE		Vitamin A	Vitamin B_1	Vitamin C	Vitamin B_2
Ordinary	Ounces	I.U. per Measure	I.U. per Measure	Milligrams per Measure	Milligrams per Measure

FRUITS *(Continued)*

Peaches, white, fresh	1 medium	4	0	5	8
" , white, canned	2 halves	3	0		4
Pears, fresh Bartlett	1 pear	3 1/5	6	5	3	0.015
Pineapple, fresh	1 slice 3/8″	1 3/5	90	13	2.6	0.006
" , canned	1 slice 3/8″	1 3/5	(90)	7	2.3
" , juice, canned	1 tumbler	6	90	35	12
Plums, fresh	2 plums	3 4/5	210	17	5.5	0.027
" , canned, not strained	2 plums	3 4/5	(200)	(15)	5
" , canned and strained	2 plums	3 4/5	(200)	(12)	2.5
Pomegranate	1 pomegranate	6	0		20
" , juice	1 tumbler	6	0			0.18
Prunes, unsulphured	4 prunes	1 2/5	350	24	trace	0.3
" , sulphured	4 prunes	1 2/5	390	0	3.9
" , stewed, unsulphured	1/2 cup		500	34	0
" , stewed, sulphured	1/2 cup		540	0	5.6
Quince	1 quince	4			11
Raisins, unsulphured	1/4 cup	1	28	21	0	0.04
" , sulphured	1/4 cup	1	28	0	0	0.04
Raspberries	1 cup	4 3/5	270	trace	33
Strawberries	1/2 box	6	340	trace	93
Tangerines	1 tangerine	2	280	22	28	0.022
Watermelon	1 slice 3/4″ x 6″ diam.	11	0	25	15	0.18

VEGETABLES*

Artichokes	1 artichoke	8 1/2	250	70	15	0.025
Asparagus, green	2 stalks 7 1/2″ long	1 1/3	130	22	19
" , bleached	2 stalks 7 1/2″ long	1 1/3	0		9
" , green, cooked, not strained	2 stalks 7 1/2″ long	1 1/3	13	22	7

*Strained vegetables are vegetables from which all the water (in cooking or in the can) has been strained off. When vegetables are pressed through a sieve, i.e., puréed, vitamins are lost unless the water is retained and used.

MEASURE		Vita-min *A*	Vita-min *B₁*	Vita-min *C*	Vita-min *B₂*
Ordinary	Ounces	*I. U. per Measure*	*I. U. per Measure*	*Milligrams per Measure*	*Milligrams per Measure*

VEGETABLES *(Continued)*

Asparagus, green, cooked, strained	2 stalks 7 1/2″ long	1 1/3	13	(3)	1
*Beans, baked, with pork	1 cup	4	15	150	0
* ″ , baked, without pork	1 cup	4	15	68	0
″ , kidney or haricot, fresh	1/2 cup	3	(27)	63	0	0.025
″ , kidney or haricot, dried	1/2 cup	3 1/2	27	70	0
″ , kidney or haricot, dried, cooked	1/2 cup	3 1/2	27	50	0
″ , navy, dried	1/2 cup	3 1/2	27	128	0
″ , navy, dried, cooked	1/2 cup	3 1/2	(27)	128	0
″ , navy, dried, cooked with soda	1/2 cup	3 1/2	(27)	128	0
″ , navy, dried, cooked, strained	1/2 cup	3 1/2	(27)	128	0
″ , lima, fresh (no pods)	1/2 cup	3	(0)	100	25	0.25
″ , lima, fresh, cooked, not strained	1/2 cup	3	(0)	100	13	0.25
″ , lima, fresh, cooked, strained	1/2 cup	3	0	75	0
″ , lima, dried	1/2 cup	2 3/4	0	92	(0)	0.25
″ , lima, dried, cooked, not strained	1/2 cup	2 3/4	0	92	(0)
″ , lima, dried, cooked, strained	1/2 cup	2 3/4		61	
″ , string or snap, green	1/2 cup	3 1/2	600	25	8	0.08
″ , string or snap, green, cooked, not strained	1/2 cup	3 1/2	600	20	7
″ , string or snap, green, cooked, strained	1/2 cup	3 1/2	600	17	4
″ , string or snap, green, cooked with soda	1/2 cup	3 1/2	600	10	
″ , string or snap, canned	1/2 cup	3 1/2	600	11	4
″ , string or snap, canned, strained	1/2 cup	3 1/2	600	11	2	0.06
″ , runner, green	1/2 cup	3 1/2	530	47	11

* These values have been calculated from typical home-cooking recipes.

MEASURE		Vitamin A	Vitamin B₁	Vitamin C	Vitamin B₂
Ordinary	Ounces	I.U. per Measure	I.U. per Measure	Milligrams per Measure	Milligrams per Measure

VEGETABLES *(Continued)*

	MEASURE	Ounces	A	B₁	C	B₂
Beans, runner, cooked, not strained	1/2 cup	3 1/2	700	(40)	(5)	
" , runner, cooked, strained	1/2 cup	3 1/2	700	(30)	(5)	
" , soy, white, dried	1/2 cup	3 1/2	140	250		
" , soy, green	1/2 cup	3 1/2		159		
" , soy, green, dried	1/2 cup	3 1/2		485	18	
" , soy, black, dried	1/2 cup	3 1/2	900	100	46	
" , wax, butter, or yellow	1/2 cup	3 1/2	410	30	16	
" , wax, butter, or yellow, cooked	1/2 cup	3 1/2	410	25		
Beets (root)	1/2 cup diced	5		70	24	5
" (root), cooked	1/2 cup diced	5		(70)	24	10
" (root), cooked, and strained	1/2 cup diced	5		(70)	(20)	5
Broccoli, fresh	1 cup	4	4000	38	80	
" , cooked, strained	1 cup	4	(4000)	25	50	
Brussels sprouts	6 sprouts 1 1/2″ diam.	4	1100	65	100	
" " , cooked, not strained	6 sprouts 1 1/2″ diam.	4	(1100)	(50)	90	
" " cooked, strained	6 sprouts 1 1/2″ diam.	4	(1100)	(25)	45	
" " , canned	6 sprouts 1 1/2″ diam.	4	(1100)	(50)	90	
" " , canned, strained	6 sprouts 1 1/2″ diam.	4	(1100)	(20)	45	
Cabbage, white, raw (English has 800 units of vitamin A per cup)						
" , white, raw, American	1 cup chopped	3 1/3	50	25	25	0.04
" , white, cooked, American (finely cut, boiled 3–15 minutes)	1 cup chopped	3 1/3	50	(20)	12	

MEASURE		Vita-min A	Vita-min B₁	Vita-min C	Vita-min B₂
Ordinary	Ounces	I. U. per Measure	I. U. per Measure	Milligrams per Measure	Milligrams per Measure

VEGETABLES *(Continued)*

Cabbage, white, cooked, American (finely cut, boiled 3–15 minutes and strained)	1 cup chopped	3 1/3	50	(10)	8
", white, cooked, American (whole leaves)	1 cup	3 1/3	50	(20)	25
", white, cooked, American (whole leaves), and strained	1 cup	3 1/3	50	(20)	12
Carrots, raw	1 cup diced	4 3/4	2700	32	8	0.03
", cooked	1 cup diced	4 3/4	2700	32	5
", cooked, strained	1 cup diced	4 3/4	(2700)	(32)	3
", canned, strained	1 cup diced	4 3/4	(2700)	13	(3)
Cauliflower	1/4 head	3	49	46	33	0.065
", cooked	1/4 head	3		(35)	33
", cooked, strained	1/4 head	3		(15)	8
Celery, green stems	2 stalks 7″ long	1 1/2	320		2
", blanched stems	2 stalks 7″ long	1 1/2	2	5	2
Chard (beet tops)	1/2 cup	5 1/5	12,000	20	43
" " " , cooked	1/2 cup	5 1/5	(12,000)	(15)	28
" " " , cooked, strained	1/2 cup	5 1/5	(12,000)	(12)	17
Chicory (escarole) green	4 leaves	3 1/2	9500		5	0.022
" " bleached	4 leaves	3 1/2	180		(4)
Chives	1 teasp.	1/5			2
Collards	1/2 cup	3 3/5	2200	68	50	0.3
", cooked	1/2 cup	3 3/5	2200	(50)	22
Corn, yellow, whole grain	1/4 cup	1 4/5	250	25	5	0.018
Corn, sweet, Country Gentleman (white)	1 ear 6″	4 1/2	125	18	4	0.13
", sweet, canned	1/2 cup	3 1/2	120	(30)	11
", Golden Bantam	1 ear 6″	4 1/2	1250	22	4
", Golden Bantam, cooked	1 ear 6″	4 1/2	1250	(15)	3
", Golden Bantam, canned	1/2 cup	3 1/2	1200	(30)	(10)

MEASURE		Vitamin A	Vitamin B_1	Vitamin C	Vitamin B_2
Ordinary	Ounces	I. U. per Measure	I. U. per Measure	Milligrams per Measure	Milligrams per Measure

VEGETABLES *(Continued)*

Cucumbers, raw	1/2 of 10″ long	6 1/2	0–20	55	18	0.003
Dandelions, greens	1 cup	3 1/2	12,500		
Eggplant	3 slices 4″ diam. 1/2″ thick	6 1/3	70	43	8	0.10
Endive	3 stalks 6″ long	7 1/3	4200	70	20
Garlic	1 clove	1/4	0		2
Kale	1 cup	3 2/5	9000	59	140	0.50
″ , cooked	1 cup	3 2/5	(9000)	45	28
Kohlrabi	1 cup 1/2″ cubes	5		16	60
″ , cooked	1 cup 1/2″ cubes	5			39
″ , cooked, strained	1 cup 1/2″ cubes	5			13
Leek	1 leek 7″ long	1	17	8 /	7
Lentils	2 tblsp.	1	25	14		0.022
″ , cooked	2 tblsp.	1	14	(10)
″ , dried	2 tblsp.	1		8
Lettuce, Romaine	2 leaves 9″ long	3/4	1300	4	1	0.03
″ , Iceberg, head	1/4 large head	2 1/2	150	20	4.5	0.05
″ , Iceberg, outer green leaves	2 large leaves	1	500	8	2	0.02
″ , Iceberg, inner head	1/4 large head	2 1/2	45	20	4.5	0.05
Mustard greens	1/2 cup	2 1/3	100	30
Okra	5 pods	2	85	23	6	0.26
Onions, spring	1 medium	2	6200
″ , fresh	1 medium	2	0–12	10	3	0.007
″ , fresh, stewed	1 medium	2	0	10
Parsley	4 stems	1/2	1000		11
Parsnips	17″ long, 2″ diam. at top	6 3/4	380	66	38
Peas, fresh	1/2 cup	2 1/3	530	85	20	0.026
″ , fresh, cooked	1/2 cup	2 1/3	530	78	13

MEASURE		Vita-min A	Vita-min B₁	Vita-min C	Vita-min B₂
Ordinary	Ounces	*I. U. per Meas-ure*	*I. U. per Meas-ure*	*Milli-grams per Meas-ure*	*Milli-grams per Meas-ure*

VEGETABLES *(Continued)*

Peas, fresh, cooked, strained	1/2 cup	2 1/3	530	68	10	
" , fresh, cooked with soda	1/2 cup	2 1/3	(530)	57		
" , canned	1/2 cup	2 1/3	(530)	79	20	
" , canned, strained	1/2 cup	2 1/3	(530)	20	6	
" , dried whole	1/2 cup	3 1/2	625	50		
" , dried whole and cooked	1/2 cup	3 1/2	(625)	30		
Peppers, green	1 pepper 3 1/2″ long	2 1/2	600	69	0.12	
Peppers, red	1 pepper 3 1/2″ long	2 1/2	2200		135	
Potatoes, yellow, sweet	1/2 medium-sized	3 3/5	8000	31	20	0.22
" , yellow, sweet, cooked	1/2 medium-sized	3 3/5	4000	(25)	10	
" , white, new	1 medium-sized	5 1/3	60	93	30	
" , white, new, cooked*	1 medium-sized	5 1/3	40	74	30	
" , white, new, cooked, strained	1 medium-sized	5 1/3	40	62	22	
" , white, canned, strained	1 cup	5 1/3	40	(60)	15	
" , white, old	1 medium-sized	5 1/3	60	73	22	
" , white, old, cooked	1 medium-sized	5 1/3	40	58	15	
" , white, old, cooked, strained	1 medium-sized	5 1/3	40	49	10	
" , white, old, baked	1 medium-sized	5 1/3	40	60	15	
Pumpkin	1/2 cup	3 1/3	190		9	0.038
Radishes	6 radishes	2	0	6	11	0.01
Rhubarb	1/2 cup 1″ pieces	2	700	trace	5.5	
" , cooked	1/2 cup 1″ pieces	2	700		1.6	
" , canned	1/2 cup 1″ pieces	2	700		0.8	

* When potatoes are cooked whole (i.e., with skins on), the loss of vitamins on cooking is very small.

MEASURE		Vitamin A	Vitamin B_1	Vitamin C	Vitamin B_2
Ordinary	Ounces	I. U. per Measure	I. U. per Measure	Milligrams per Measure	Milligrams per Measure

VEGETABLES *(Continued)*

Rutabagas	1 cup 1/2″ cubes	5	10	28	22	0.13

		Vit A	Vit B1	Vit C	Vit B2
Rutabagas — 1 cup 1/2″ cubes	5	10	28	22	0.13
Sauerkraut, fresh — 1 cup	5			16	
″ , bulk, commercial — 1 cup	5		trace	10	
″ , cooked — 1 cup	5			3	
″ , canned — 1 cup	5			9	
″ , juice, fresh — 2 tblsp.	1			4	
″ , juice, old — 2 tblsp.	1			1	
Spinach — 1/2 cup chopped	3 3/5	14,000	37	53	0.065
″ , cooked — 1/2 cup chopped	3 3/5	(14,000)	30	26	
″ , cooked, strained — 1/2 cup chopped	3 3/5	(14,000)	27	13	
″ , canned, strained — 1 cup	3 3/5	(12,000)	7	13	
Squash, winter, Hubbard — 1/2 cup	4	2900	21	3.5	
″ , summer — 1/2 cup	4	170	16	(3.5)	
Tapioca — 2 tblsp.	1	0	0	0	0
Tomatoes — 1 medium	7	6000	52	50	0.10
″ , canned — 1/2 cup	4 1/4	3600	25	24	
″ , canned, strained — 1/2 cup	4 1/4	3600	(15)	(15)	
″ , juice, canned — 1 tumbler	6	5300	25	25	
Turnip greens — 1/2 cup	3	6000	38	42	0.25
″ ″ , cooked — 1/2 cup	3	(6000)	25	10	
″ root — 1 cup 1/2″ pieces	5 1/2	0	30	31	0.062
″ ″ , cooked — 1 cup 1/2″ pieces	5 1/2	0	trace	26	
″ ″ , cooked, strained — 1 cup 1/2″ pieces	5 1/2	0		20	
Watercress — 1/2 bunch	1 1/2	2000	28	22	

NUTS

		Vit A	Vit B1	Vit C	Vit B2
Almonds — 10 nuts	3/5	0	7	0.5	
Cashew — 5 nuts	1/2	19			0.028
Chestnuts — 2 nuts	1/2		12	5	
Coconut, shredded, fresh — 1 tblsp.	1/3	0	1	0.5	0.014

	MEASURE		Vita-min A	Vita-min B_1	Vita-min C	Vita-min B_2
	Ordinary	Ounces	I. U. per Meas-ure	I. U. per Meas-ure	Milli-grams per Meas-ure	Milli-grams per Meas-ure

NUTS *(Continued)*

Coconut, milk, fresh	1 cup	8	0	0	4	
Hazel	10 nuts	1/2		28	2	
Peanuts, whole, Spanish, shelled	1/3 cup	1 1/2	17	146	4	0.3
" , whole, Spanish, shelled, roasted	1/3 cup	1 1/2		33	0	
" , Virginia type, shelled	1/3 cup	1 1/2	17	105	4	0.3
Peanut butter	2 tblsp.	1 1/2	17	125		
Pecans	12 nuts	1/2	14			
Pistachio	15 nuts	1/2	55			
Walnuts	12 nuts	1/2	190	16	3.5	

MISCELLANEOUS

Corn oil			0	0	0	0
Cottonseed oil			0	0	0	0
*Ice cream, home-made with cream	serving	8	925	25	3	
*Ice cream, commercial, made with skim milk	serving	8	0	15	3	
Lard			0	0	0	0
*Mayonnaise	1 tblsp.		30	0.5	0	
Molasses, tinned, commercial			0	trace	0	0
Oleomargarine (unless vitamin A added)			0	0	0	0
Olive oil			trace	0	0	0
*Pie, apple	1 serving		90	14	0	
* " , blueberry	1 serving		62	9	3	
* " , chocolate meringue	1 serving		440	10	0.5	
Sago			0	0	0	0
*Soup, black bean	1 cup	4	70	11	0	
* " , split pea	1 cup	4	145	18	0	
* " , tomato	1 cup	4	1480	10	9	
* " , vegetable	1 cup	4	276	9	4	
Sugar			0	0	0	
Tea, as beverage			0	0	0	0
Coffee, as beverage			0	0	0	0

* These values have been calculated from typical home-cooking recipes.

MEASURE		Vita-min A	Vita-min B_1	Vita-min C	Vita-min B_2
Ordinary	Ounces	*I. U. per Meas-ure*	*I. U. per Meas-ure*	*Milli-grams per Meas-ure*	*Milli-grams per Meas-ure*

MISCELLANEOUS *(Continued)*

Cocoa	2 tblsp.	1/2	0	4	0	0
Beer	1 glass	6	0	4	0	0
Yeast, baker's, compressed	1 cake	2	0	100	1	1.4
" , baker's, dried	1 cake	1/2	0	70		0.5
" , brewer's, fresh	1 cake	2	100	220		0.85
" , brewer's, dried	1 cake	1/2		80–500		0.4

Index